Endocrinology

THIRD EDITION

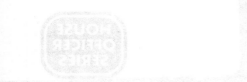

Endocrinology

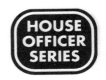

Endocrinology

THIRD EDITION

Warner M. Burch, M.D.

Associate Professor
Departments of Medicine and Pharmacology
Duke University Medical Center
Durham, North Carolina

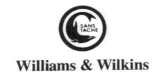

Williams & Wilkins

BALTIMORE • PHILADELPHIA • HONG KONG
LONDON • MUNICH • SYDNEY • TOKYO

A WAVERLY COMPANY

Editor: Timothy S. Satterfield
Managing Editor: Linda S. Napora
Copy Editor: Therese J. Grundl
Designer: Dan Pfisterer
Illustration Planner: Ray Lowman
Production Coordinator: Charles E. Zeller

Copyright © 1994
Williams & Wilkins
428 East Preston Street
Baltimore, Maryland 21202, USA

Accurate indications, adverse reactions, and dosage schedules for drugs are provided in this book, but it is possible that they may change. The reader is urged to review the package information data of the manufacturers of the medications mentioned.

Printed in the United States of America

First Edition 1984   Second Edition 1988

Library of Congress Cataloging in Publication Data
Burch, Warner M.
   Endocrinology for the house officer / Warner M. Burch.—3rd ed.
       p.   cm. — (House officer series)
   Includes bibliographical references and index.
   ISBN 0-683-01131-6
   1. Endocrine glands—Diseases—Handbooks, manuals, etc.
  2. Endocrinology—Handbooks, manuals, etc.   I. Title.   II. Series.
   [DNLM: 1. Endocrine Diseases—handbooks. WK 39 B947e 1994]
   RC648.B87   1994
616.4—dc20
DNLM/DLC
for Library of Congress   93-4721
                                                                   CIP
                                                                    98
                                        4   5   6   7   8   9 10

About the Author

Warner M. Burch, M.D., a graduate of Wake Forest College, attended Bowman Gray School of Medicine. After a rotating internship at Charlotte Memorial Hospital, Dr. Burch completed his medicine residency and fellowship in endocrinology at Duke University Medical Center. While in the military, he taught students in United States Navy and Air Force Physicians' Assistants Programs. Dr. Burch holds the rank of Associate Professor of Medicine and Assistant Professor of Pharmacology. He wrote the companion book, *Case Studies in Endocrinology for the House Officer,* also published by Williams & Wilkins.

Preface

Endocrinology in the House Officer Series addresses endocrine problems commonly encountered in medical practice. The third edition is different from the first two: each chapter has been expanded, and the publisher, instead of the author, designed and formatted the text. Its approach is still the same: largely problem-oriented with emphasis on workup, diagnosis, and treatment. It is not intended to be a textbook of endocrinology but a convenient and practical "how to" and "why" source that can be used on the wards and in the clinic. The author would appreciate any feedback and tips that might be included in future revisions. We all remain students of medicine and servants to others.

Warner M. Burch, M.D.

Acknowledgments

Writing a book requires time and support from many people, mostly patients who continue to teach me and a family who put up with my "nose in the computer." I thank the many physicians who helped make this a useful book.

Contents

Chapter 1

Endocrine Tests

WHEN, HOW, AND WHAT THEY MEAN

Probably nothing is more confusing than the myriad endocrine studies available to physicians. There are numerous studies, but only those that are widely available will be discussed in this chapter. As with any laboratory study, a clinical diagnosis or intuition from the history or physical examination will lead one to order a particular study. What to do with the laboratory results can be a problem. An ideal test would always give positive results in anyone with disease and negative results in anyone without disease. There would be no false-positive or false-negative results. However, no such test meets these standards. Three factors must be integrated into the interpretation of a test result: sensitivity, specificity, and prevalence of the disorder in question. A good test is positive in disease (sensitivity) and negative in health (specificity). For example, a urine study that identifies elevated catecholamines in 95 of 100 patients with pheochromocytoma has 95% sensitivity. If the same urine study is performed in 100 healthy volunteers and 99 of the values are normal, then the test has 99% specificity. How well a test performs can be stated in its predictive value. The predictive value of a positive test (percentage of all positive results that are truly positive) depends significantly on the prevalence of the underlying disorder. Prevalence, probably the most important and least appreciated factor, dramatically affects the usefulness of a test result (Table 1.1). The striking effect of prevalence can be demonstrated using a superior test with 99% sensitivity and 99% specificity (something that is rare in clinical medicine). If the prevalence of the disorder is 1 in a 1000, then there is only a 9% probability that a positive test result is truly positive (i.e., 91% false-positive result).

Often, a new test looks great, but when it is applied in clinical practice failure and disillusion follow. Typically, an investigator de-

Table 1.1
**Effect of Prevalence on Predictive Value When
Sensitivity and Specificity Equal 99%**

Prevalence (%)	Predictive Value of a Positive Test (%)
0.1	9.0
1.0	50.0
2.0	66.9
5.0	83.9
50.0	99.0

velops a test in which 100 subjects with a disease (e.g., hypothyroidism) are tested, and the results detect 99 of the 100 patients with
hypothyroidism (sensitivity 99%). Another 100 patients (laboratory
personnel, medical students, paid volunteers) are tested who are clinically euthyroid. Only one of the 100 has a positive result (specificity
99%). The investigator publishes a paper extolling the virtues of the
test. Later, the hospital laboratory offers the test screening for hypothyroidism. Other physicians find that some patients coming for
elective surgery have positive results; some patients on medications
have positive results, and patients with acute disease have positive results. Few of these actually are hypothyroid. What happened?

The investigator and reviewers forgot that prevalence may be
more important than sensitivity and specificity. When the investigator
studied the original 200 subjects (100 with and 100 without hypothyroidism), the disease prevalence was 50%! The predictive value of a
positive test would be 99% (Table 1.1). When the test was applied to
all hospital admissions, the test did not change, only the prevalence of
the disease. If the prevalence dropped to 1 of 100, the predictive value
of the test would be 50%, meaning that half of the positive tests would
be false-positive. If hypothyroidism occurred in 1 in 1000 (as in outpatients), then screening *all* subjects with the same test would have a
predictive value of 9%, meaning 91 of 100 patients with positive tests
would have a false result. The job of the clinician is to order studies in
patients who are likely to have the disease (increasing the prevalence);
then a positive result is more likely to be a true positive.

When there is discordance between clinical diagnosis and laboratory results, then the laboratory may be in error. Somehow clinicians
have been "sold a bill of goods" regarding the infallibility of a laboratory result. If your clinical diagnosis seems firm yet the results dis-

agree, then contact the laboratory: ask for a repeat run; check if the proper patient sample was assayed; check how good that assay was; and so forth. With endocrine studies in general, it is very important that you know the quality and reliability of the laboratory to which the specimen was sent. This point cannot be overemphasized.

THYROID TESTS
Serum Thyroxine

The most widely used method for measuring total serum thyroxine (T4) is the radioimmunoassay (RIA). It is reliable, inexpensive, and specific. Normal serum T4(RIA) levels range between 5 and 12 μg/dL. Serum T4 is affected by two major factors: <u>thyroid secretion of T4</u> and the <u>serum binding capacity for T4</u>. Because >99.9% of the T4 circulating is bound to protein, any alteration in the binding capacity as well as in T4 secretion leads to abnormal serum T4 levels. To accurately interpret the level of T4, one must know about the serum T4 binding capacity. The following case illustrates a common situation. A 24-year woman was referred because of symptoms of anxiety and rapid heart rate; her serum T4(RIA) was 14.5 μg/dL (normal 5–12). She was taking an oral contraceptive. On physical examination the pulse was 95/minute, and no goiter was palpated. Is this hyperthyroidism? Unlikely, but what one really needs is a measure of the serum T4 binding capacity because estrogens increase thyroid binding globulin (TBG), the major T4 binding serum protein. The T4 binding capacity of serum is assessed by measuring the thyroid hormone binding index or ratio (T3U).

T3U or Triiodothyronine Resin Uptake

T3U measures indirectly the number of unoccupied protein binding sites for T4 and triiodothyronine (T3) in serum. The test gets its name from the radiolabeled T3 used in the in vitro assay. Radiolabeled T3 is added to the patient's serum and competes for binding sites on the TBG molecule. Radiolabeled T3 is used instead of T4 because the assay time is shorter. A resin or some other inert material is then added to adsorb any unbound radiolabeled T3. The radioactivity of the resin is then counted and expressed as percent of total counts added to the assay tube. If the sites on TBG are underoccupied by T4 (as in hypothyroidism with decreased T4 secretion), then more radiolabeled T3 binds to the protein and less radiolabeled T3 is adsorbed to the resin. Thus the T3U is low. In patients with hyperthyroidism (increased T4 secretion), the T3U is elevated since most of the sites on TBG are occupied by T4 so that less radiolabeled T3 can be bound by the protein and more to the resin. The normal range of values for the T3U depends on the particular type of resin used, which means various laboratories have different normal ranges for T3U. When TBG levels are raised (i.e., more binding sites for radiolabeled T3, less radioactivity for resin to adsorb), the T3U will be low. In all cases, however, the T3U is inversely proportional to the number of unoccupied binding sites on TBG (low T3U—high TBG; high T3U—low TBG). Estrogen, the most frequent medication that raises TBG, does so by decreasing the hepatic clearance of TBG.

The patient mentioned above who was taking an oral contraceptive had raised TBG levels that were confirmed with a low T3U. There are numerous factors that may affect TBG and thus the T3U value. These factors are listed in Table 1.2.

Some medications, such as salicylates (high doses), phenytoin, and clofibrate, compete with T4 to bind on TBG. This leads to high T3U values but also to lower T4(RIA) levels. <u>Remember that the T3U has nothing to do with the serum levels of T3.</u>

To correct for variation in TBG (and therefore the T4 and T3U values), a calculated value called the <u>free thyroid index</u> may be used. The free thyroid index is an attempt to normalize discordant serum T4 and T3U values and is the product of the T4(RIA) times the T3U. This calculated number correlates well with the levels of free T4 and thus is named free thyroid index.

Table 1.2
Effect of TBG on T3U Values

Increased TBG; T3U low	Decreased TBG; T3U high
Estrogen therapy	Androgen therapy
Pregnancy	Severe hypoproteinemia
Acute hepatitis	Chronic liver disease
Acute intermittent porphyria	Glucocorticoid excess
Hereditary TBG increase	Hereditary TBG deficiency
	Acromegaly

Free Thyroxine

The unbound or free T4 is the metabolically active hormone fraction. It accounts for <0.05% of the total T4 circulating in the blood. Ideally, the measurement of the free T4 would eliminate most of the confusion regarding binding protein abnormalities because it circulates within well-defined limits in the euthyroid patient. Free T4 levels have not been routinely available because the measurement of this small quantity of unbound T4 is technically difficult, time consuming, and often requires dialysis techniques for quantitation. However, the commercial kits for measurement of free T4 have improved considerably. If one uses radiolabeled T4 derivatives that do not bind significantly to TBG and high affinity antibodies that bind both T4 and T4 derivative, then a classical equilibrium RIA can be applied. This technology gives reliable free T4 values and promises to replace T4(RIA).

Triiodothyronine

The primary hormone secreted and the major circulating thyroid hormone is T4. However, T4 is rapidly deiodinated into T3 by 5'-deiodinase found in many tissues but especially in the liver. T3, the metabolically active thyroid hormone, binds to nuclear receptors of target tissues. T3 circulates in the blood at concentrations 50 times lower than T4. RIAs of T3 are specific and are generally available. Serum T3(RIA) levels range between 90 and 190 ng/dL. T3 is also bound to TBG, but the affinity is less avid. Nevertheless, serum T3(RIA) measurements are subject to the same limitations regarding protein binding as are T4 determinations (e.g., estrogens increase TBG and therefore raise T3(RIA) levels). Serum T3(RIA) levels are elevated in hyperthyroidism, often to a greater degree than the T4(RIA). Serum T3(RIA) is useful in iodine deficient states where the T4 may be low yet the T3 normal. T3(RIA) is particularly useful in hyperthyroid states such as toxic nodular goiter where the serum T4 may be normal. Free T3 determinations are commercially available using techniques comparable with free T4 measurements described above.

Thyroid-Stimulating Hormone

Levels of thyroid-stimulating hormone (TSH), a glycoprotein secreted by the pituitary, depend on the concentration of circulating free T4. This is a classic negative feedback system. Low levels of T4 lead to

TSH secretion that stimulates thyroid hormone production and release which in turn decrease pituitary TSH output. Conversely, high T4 or T3 levels suppress TSH secretion. In fact, a log-linear relationship exists between TSH and free T4; a 2-fold decline in free T4 concentration is accompanied by a 160-fold increase in TSH concentrations. Current TSH assays using immunoradiometric or immunochemiluminometric assays are sensitive enough to tell the difference between 0 and 2 μU/mL, which older assays could not do. Current assays use a "sandwich" technique in which a monoclonal antibody is prepared against the α-chain of TSH and a different monoclonal prepared against the β-chain. One antibody is tagged with 125-iodine or an acridinium ester depending on the assay type (immunoradiometric or immunochemiluminometric, respectively). The other monoclonal is attached to an inert surface (e.g., coated tube or plastic bead). Serum is incubated with these antibodies. One portion of TSH binds to the inert surface and another portion binds to the labeled antibody. After washing away the unbound labeled antibody, the bound tracer is counted. The hormone is sandwiched between the antibodies, permitting great specificity and uncanny sensitivity particularly with immunochemiluminometric assay. Furthermore, this technique allows one to measure hormones (adrenocorticotropic hormone (ACTH) and parathyroid hormone (PTH)) for which reliable levels have been difficult to obtain. The improved sensitivity allows differentiation between euthyroid and hyperthyroid subjects whose TSH levels are low (0–0.2 μU/mL). Serum TSH in healthy subjects ranges from 0.4 to 6 μU/mL with the mean between 1 and 2 μU/mL. The serum TSH is elevated in primary hypothyroidism usually over 20 μU/mL, reaching levels >100 μU/mL. <u>Measuring TSH is the best single thyroid test to screen for thyroid function in outpatients.</u>

Thyrotropin-Releasing Hormone

Thyrotropin-releasing hormone (TRH), a tripeptide secreted by the hypothalamus, reaches the pituitary via the portal-hypophyseal capillary system. TRH stimulates target pituitary cells (thyrotropes) to secrete TSH. If ambient levels of T4 or T3 are high, then the thyrotrope does not respond to TRH with a rise in TSH. In primary hypothyroidism in which TSH levels are already elevated, TRH greatly augments the release of TSH. TRH administration is useful when hyperthyroidism is suspected but has been replaced almost exclusively by the sensitive TSH assay. Giving TRH provides a dynamic test that assesses the functional integrity of the thyrotrope. The <u>TRH study</u> is performed as follows. **Blood is drawn for baseline TSH (0 time). TRH (protirelin) 500 μg iv is given over 15–20 seconds and blood drawn again at 30 minutes for TSH determination. TSH levels peak normally around 20–30 minutes after TRH. The normal response depends on age and sex. Females generally have at least a 6-μU/mL rise above the basal level. Males younger than 40 years should have a similar rise (>6 μU/mL), whereas males >40 should have at least a 2 μU/ mL rise.** In primary hypothyroidism the response to TRH is increased. Hyperthyroid patients, patients with euthyroid Graves' disease, or subjects taking excessive doses of replacement thyroid (T4 or T3) or pharmacological amounts of glucocorticoid fail to produce a rise in serum TSH.

Thyroidal 24-Hour Radioactive Iodine Uptake

The thyroid gland concentrates iodine that it uses for T4 production. Because the thyroid acts as a sump for iodine and relatively little iodine is trapped anywhere else in the body, the uptake of radioactive iodine (RAI) is a useful marker of thyroid function. The source of radioactivity has traditionally been 131-iodine. The RAI uptake is calculated as the percentage of total administered radioactivity taken up by the thyroid. This determination is usually made 24 hours after an oral ingestion of tracer doses of 131-iodine (6–8 μCi). The normal 24-hour RAI uptake is 10–30%.

If the thyroid is not functioning (e.g., hypothyroidism or in subacute thyroiditis where the follicular cells cannot concentrate iodine), then the 24-hour RAI uptake is low. If the iodine content of the plasma pool is elevated secondary to ingestion of iodine-rich foods (kelp) or medications (saturated solution of potassium iodide, amiodarone, etc.) or secondary to the administration of radiographic agents, then the 24-hour value for tracer uptake is low even though the thyroid may function normally.

In diffuse toxic goiter the thyroidal trapping of iodine is increased, and the 24-hour 131-iodine uptake will be elevated. 123-Iodine is now a frequent source of RAI since there is less radiation exposure to the thyroid. The amount of radiation delivered to the thyroid by 131-iodine is approximately 1.5 rad/μCi (assuming normal size gland and 20% 24-hr uptake), which is 100 times the radiation exposure of 123-iodine (0.015 rad/μCi). <u>All radionuclide tests are contraindicated during pregnancy.</u>

Thyroid Imaging or Scan

Imaging of the thyroid is possible by utilizing radionuclides. These are useful in ascertaining whether a particular area of the thyroid, such as a nodule, is functioning, i.e., can it trap and concentrate the radionuclide? The most often used radiotracers are <u>technetium-99m pertechnetate (TcO4-99m)</u>, <u>131-iodine</u>, and <u>123-iodine</u>. TcO4-99m (5 mCi) is administrated intravenously, and thyroid imaging is performed within 30 minutes. TcO4-99m assesses only the transport ability of the follicular cells, whereas iodine radionuclides assess both transport and organification of iodine to thyroglobulin. The amount of radiation delivered to the thyroid is 0.2 rad/mCi TcO4-99m. 131-Iodine (50 μCi) is administrated orally and the scan performed 24 hours later. The thyroid scan with pertechnetate is more convenient for the patient and also has considerably less thyroidal radiation (i.e., 1 rad vs 75 rad for 131-iodine). 123-Iodine may also be used for imaging. This isotope is not always readily available because of its short half-life (13 hours).

PITUITARY TESTS
Growth hormone

Growth hormone (GH) is measured in three circumstances: (*a*) when there is clinical evidence of <u>acromegaly or gigantism</u>, (*b*) when there is evidence of <u>growth failure</u> (e.g., short stature), and (*c*) when it is necessary to ascertain whether there is <u>adequate pituitary reserve</u>. Mass lesions (e.g., tumors, cysts) often impair GH secretion by the pituitary somatotrope, making GH levels a sensitive marker of deranged pituitary function. GH is assayed in serum or plasma using RIA. A single determination of GH can be useful in a few cases, but often dynamic studies (stimulation or suppression tests) are necessary.

If the question is <u>acromegaly</u>, obtain a blood sample after the patient has fasted overnight and is at bed rest. A GH level of >10 ng/mL is highly suggestive of acromegaly. Any form of stress (exercise, surgery, smoking, etc.) raises GH, and thus caution must be taken on borderline elevated values. Because rises in blood glucose suppress GH levels in healthy patients, acromegaly is usually confirmed using an oral glucose tolerance test (see Chapter 3). Blood is obtained at 0, 60, 120, and 180 minutes for GH determination. Normal subjects exhibit a decrease in GH to <2 ng/mL within 2 hours. Up to one-third of acromegalic patients have a paradoxical rise in GH levels during the glucose tolerance test. GH stimulates somatomedin production, so <u>insulin-like growth factor I</u> levels are elevated in acromegaly as well.

If the question is <u>GH deficiency</u>, then one determination using any form of stress to raise GH may be all that is necessary. In children, blood drawn for GH 90 minutes after sleep is helpful because GH is secreted during REM sleep. However, a more practical study is to have the child exercise (run up and down steps for 15 minutes) and then draw blood for GH level. Any values above 5 ng/mL exclude GH deficiency. Various stimulatory tests are available to raise GH levels. Determining when to order these studies and how to interpret them requires discernment. In short children with low GH values after exercise or in patients with possible hypopituitarism, a stimulatory test or dynamic study is indicated.

The "gold standard" dynamic study is insulin-induced hypoglycemia. Hypoglycemia produces a profound stress reaction that is followed by GH and ACTH release, with a subsequent rise in the serum cortisol. **The <u>insulin-induced hypoglycemia test</u> is performed in the morning after an overnight fast with the patient at bed rest. An indwelling needle in the forearm is recommended so that multiple samples can be obtained. Blood for basal levels of GH and cortisol is taken at -15 and 0 minutes. Regular insulin (0.1 U/kg for normal-sized patients and 0.15–0.2 U/kg for patients with insulin resistance, e.g., obesity) is injected as an intravenous bolus over 10–15 seconds. If there is clinical evidence of hypopituitarism, then a lower dose of insulin is used (0.05 U/kg), since profound hypoglycemia is more likely. Plasma glucose is measured at 0, 15, 30, 45, and 60 minutes. A decrease of the plasma glucose to 50% of the baseline value *or* <40 mg/dL is considered an adequate hypoglycemic response, which is necessary to interpret the GH and cortisol levels. Blood for GH and cortisol is measured at 0, 30, 60, and 90 minutes. Dextrose (50%) should be available to treat severe hypoglycemia (e.g., obtundation, seizure).** After hypoglycemia is assured (hunger, palpitations, perspiration), the patient may drink fruit juice to decrease symptoms if necessary. The nadir for the blood sugar is usually 20–30 minutes, with rises of GH and cortisol later (Fig. 1.1).

Even though sugar may have to be given intravenously or per os, continue to draw blood at the indicated intervals. GH levels normally rise to >9 ng/mL 60–90 minutes after insulin injection. The disadvantages of insulin-induced hypoglycemia are obvious: close monitor-

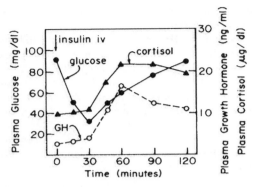

Figure 1.1. Response of plasma GH and cortisol to insulin-induced hypoglycemia.

ing of the patient is a necessity; hypoglycemia is uncomfortable, and potential problems are very real; it is not easily performed in children; and one must be sure of adequate hypoglycemia (stress) to have a valid study. In addition up to 20% of normal subjects have an impaired or absent GH response to this gold standard. Patients with obesity, Cushing's syndrome, and chronic renal failure may also have an impaired or absent GH response. However, a normal response excludes GH deficiency. Other GH stimulatory studies include oral L-dopa and arginine infusion for adults, and oral clonidine and intramuscular glucagon for children.

ACTH or Corticotropin

Because there are abundant numbers of corticotrope cells dispersed throughout the pituitary, ACTH is generally the last tropic hormone lost in pituitary disease. Normal ACTH levels range between 9 and 52 pg/mL. The method of collection and handling of the plasma sample is critical. Since ACTH adheres to glass avidly, blood must be collected, stored on ice, and centrifuged within 30 minutes (preferably earlier) and then the plasma stored at $-20°C$ in polypropylene vials. Current ACTH assays using the "sandwich" technique are quite good. Plasma ACTH levels are elevated in primary adrenal insufficiency (where serum cortisol is low). Plasma ACTH is useful in separating the types of Cushing's syndrome, particularly in ectopic ACTH where levels are often very high (>400 pg/mL) and in patients with adrenal adenoma where ACTH levels are nonmeasurable. However, ACTH levels alone do not analyze the pituitary-adrenal axis. This axis can be assessed by measuring the end-product (glucocorticoids) in a 24-hour urine collection for either 17-hydroxycorticosteroids (17-OHCS) or free cortisol (UC). Normal urinary 17-OHCS levels range between 2 and 6.5 mg/g creatinine. UC values depend on the method and the specificity of the antibody. Thus normal ranges must be established in each laboratory.

Stimulatory tests to indirectly evaluate ACTH reserve include <u>cosyntropin stimulation</u>, <u>insulin-induced hypoglycemia test</u>, and <u>metyrapone loading</u>. Ideally, the hypothalamic hormone, corticotropin-releasing hormone, could be used to assess corticotrope reserve, but its nonavailability to most physicians limits its use. The information gained from these studies is helpful in deciding whether patients have pituitary disease or whether those with known pituitary dysfunction (e.g., after pituitary surgery) need long-term glucocorticoid coverage.

Cosyntropin Stimulation

Loss of ACTH causes adrenal cortical atrophy. ACTH stimulates adrenal steroidogenesis that maintains adrenal volume and weight. This preservation of adrenal mass is quite sensitive to and dependent on ACTH. For example, after 2–4 weeks of administering excessive steroids, adrenal weight loss is considerable, and cortical atrophy can be demonstrated. This loss of adrenal function can be assessed biochemically by measuring serum cortisol after administration of synthetic ACTH (cosyntropin). **Blood is taken at 0 time. Cosyntropin 0.25 mg im (or iv) is given. Another plasma cortisol is obtained at 60 minutes. Normal subjects respond to cosyntropin by raising their plasma cortisol to $\geq$18 μg/dL** (Fig. 1.2). The cosyntropin study is convenient and easily performed in an outpatient setting. Its major drawback is that it indirectly assesses pituitary function. For patients who have been hypopituitary for weeks to months, the cosyntropin study is valid. Failure to respond establishes hypopituitarism (secondary hypoadrenalism). For those who may have recently become hypoadrenal over the last 2–4 weeks from hypopituitarism (e.g., pituitary apoplexy), a normal cosyntropin study would not exclude hypoadrenalism because the adrenal glands had not enough time to atrophy. I use this study 95% of the time to assess the pituitary-adrenal axis.

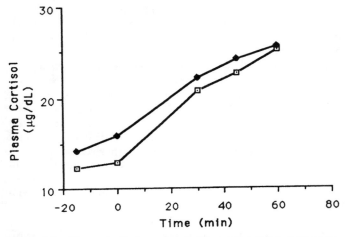

Figure 1.2. Plasma cortisol response in 10 normal subjects given cosyntropin 0.25 mg iv (*open squares*) or im (*solid diamonds*) in a double-blinded crossover study. Route of administration did not affect plasma cortisol response.

Insulin-Induced Hypoglycemia Study

Hypoglycemia is a potent stress. Utilizing the insulin-induced hypoglycemia is an excellent method to gather GH and cortisol data to assess the integrity of the pituitary-adrenal axis. Plasma cortisols are measured at the intervals listed above in the insulin-induced hypoglycemia test. Plasma cortisol should rise to a value of >18 μg/dL in normal subjects (Fig. 1.1). This study assumes the adrenal glands are intact to respond to ACTH. Since hypoglycemia is potentially life-threatening to the hypoadrenal patient, this study should be avoided in patients with known Addison's disease.

Metyrapone Loading

Metyrapone inhibits the final enzymatic step (11-β-hydroxylase) in the synthesis of cortisol, leading to a build-up of 11-deoxycortisol, the immediate precursor of cortisol, and to a decrease in cortisol production. The pituitary corticotropes sense the fall in serum cortisol levels and respond by increasing ACTH production in the fashion of the classical negative feedback loop. Although serum deoxycortisol levels rise, the pituitary does not recognize deoxycortisol as a glucocorticoid hormone. As a result, administration of metyrapone leads to elevated levels of deoxycortisol and low, normal, or raised serum cortisol (the absolute levels of cortisol depend on the effectiveness of the metyrapone-induced blockade). Metyrapone is usually administrated orally using either of the following protocols: an abbreviated overnight study or the classic 3-day study. **In the overnight study, metyrapone (3 g or 30 mg/kg) is taken at bedtime with milk to avoid gastric irritation. Since metyrapone decreases serum cortisol at the time (early morning) when the corticotrope is most sensitive to falling cortisol levels, there is an exaggerated ACTH output that leads to elevated levels of serum deoxycortisol. At 7–8 AM blood is drawn for deoxycortisol and cortisol levels. The normal response is >7 μg/dL for serum deoxycortisol. Serum cortisol levels should be low (<5 μg/dL) to assure that metyrapone produced an adequate blockade. If there is a normal deoxycortisol response, no further study is needed to assess the pituitary-adrenal axis.** If abnormal, then the 3-day protocol is performed because it is the gold standard of the metyrapone studies. **Urine is collected for 24 hours as baseline for determination of 17-OHCS (day 1). Metyrapone is given 750 mg po every 4 hours for six doses (day 2). Again metyrapone blocks cortisol production that in turn normally stimulates ACTH and deoxycortisol production. Because both cortisol and deoxycortisol have the 17,21-dihydroxyl, 20-keto groups that are measured as Porter-Silber chromatogens in the 17-OHCS assay, urine 17-OHCS levels should rise. A 24-hour urine is collected on day 3 (day after oral metyrapone). A normal rise in urine 17-OHCS is 2.5 to 3 times the baseline day's 17-OHCS value.** Table 1.3 lists a protocol for ordering this metyrapone study.

One measures the 17-OHCS level on the day after metyrapone because the last two doses of metyrapone given on day 2 produce the lowest cortisol levels (early morning) that stimulate ACTH, and thus steroidogenesis is reflected in the large amount of 17-OHCS in the subsequent collection. It is important not to give any exogenous glucocorticoid (small doses of dexamethasone) "to cover" the patient during any metyrapone study because this will inhibit ACTH release (as cortisol does), and therefore no effect on adrenosteroidogenesis will be seen.

Both insulin-induced hypoglycemia and metyrapone blockade are artificial forms of stress. Although ACTH reserve may be adequate by these studies, the question remains whether patients can handle stress

Table 1.3
Protocol for Metyrapone Loading Study

Day 1   Collect 24-hour urine (7 AM–7 AM) for 17-OHCS
Day 2   Blood draw at 7 AM for plasma cortisol and deoxycortisol
        Metyrapone 750 mg po every 4 hours for six doses (start giving
            medication at 8 AM)
        Collect 24-hour urine (7 AM–7 AM) for 17-OHCS
Day 3   Blood draw at 7 AM for plasma cortisol and deoxycortisol
        Collect 24-hour urine (7 AM–7 AM) for 17-OHCS

---

in real situations (severe infections, myocardial infarction, major surgery, etc.). Generally, if one of these studies demonstrates adequate ACTH-cortisol reserve, then no steroid coverage is necessary.

Dexamethasone suppression studies are performed whenever there is evidence of glucocorticoid excess (obesity, hypertension, protein catabolism, etc.) and the patient is not taking exogenous steroids (the most common cause of Cushing's syndrome). The study is based on the observation that small doses of a potent glucocorticosteroid (dexamethasone) inhibit the normal pituitary corticotrope so that no ACTH is released (the typical negative feedback loop), and thus there is decreased production of cortisol. Because the amount of dexamethasone does not interfere with the assay of cortisol or 17-OHCS, there is a fall of serum cortisol that is reflected in low urine cortisol and urine 17-OHCS levels. There are several ways to administer the dexamethasone.

A short overnight study is useful in the outpatient setting to screen for glucocorticoid excess (Cushing's syndrome). Dexamethasone 1 mg po is taken between 11 PM and midnight, and a serum cortisol is drawn between 8 and 9 AM the next morning. This level should be ≤ 3 μg/dL. If the serum cortisol is >3 μg/mL, then various possibilities exist: Cushing's syndrome; patient did not take dexamethasone; stress during the night; traffic rush getting to clinic; patient is pregnant or taking medications such as estrogens that increase cortisol-binding globulin; the patient is taking anticonvulsant drugs that speed metabolism of dexamethasone so that adequate suppressive levels are not reached; severe mental depression; and obesity.

A 24-hour urine for cortisol determination (UC) should be collected (see "Adrenal Tests") if the plasma cortisol is not suppressed with overnight dexamethasone. Alternatively, one can obtain a 24-hour urine for UC to screen for Cushing's syndrome and forego the overnight dexathasone study. If the UC is elevated, then the diagnosis of hypercortisolism is confirmed. Many protocols are available to define the etiology of Cushing's syndrome. I prefer Liddle's test using dexamethasone suppression of urine 17-OHCS and let the patient (if competent) collect urine as an outpatient. **This classic study is performed as follows. Two baseline 24-hour urines are collected for 17-OHCS and UC (days 1 and 2). Normal urine 17-OHCS is <6.5 mg/g creatinine, and UC is <100 μg/24 hours. Dexamethasone 0.5 mg po is given every 6 hours for eight doses (days 3 and 4), and a 24-hour urine is collected on day 4 for 17-OHCS and UC. This amount of dexamethasone (low dose: 2 mg/day) suppresses the normal corticotrope, but in patients with Cushing's syndrome (any state of hypercortisolism) the 24-hour urine does not suppress to <2.5 mg 17-OHCS/g creatinine or <25 μg cortisol/24 hours. In Cushing's disease (pituitary-dependent adrenal hyperplasia) the abnormal corticotropes in the pituitary adenoma are <u>sensitive to glucocorticoid inhibition only at much higher doses of dexamethasone</u>. Thus dexamethasone 2.0 mg po is given every 6 hours for eight doses (days 5 and 6), and a 24-hour urine is collected on day 6 for 17-OHCS determination. With this high dose of dexamethasone (8 mg/day), patients with Cushing's disease have urine 17-OHCS below 50% of the baseline values of days 1 and 2 (Fig. 1.3), whereas patients with hypercortisolism caused by adrenal adenoma/carcinoma or ectopic ACTH syndrome have no suppression of the 17-OHCS.** The reliability of the >50% criteria for sup-

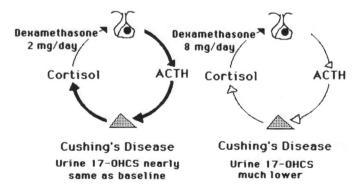

Figure 1.3.   Effect of oral dexamethasone in Cushing's disease.

pression in Cushing's disease is somewhat arbitrary because some patients with Cushing's disease may only suppress 35%. The point is that there is significant lowering of urine 17-OHCS with high dose dexamethasone in pituitary-dependent adrenal hyperplasia (see page 95 for further discussion).

Others have used modifications of the high dose dexamethasone study to shorten the workup. At 8 AM a baseline plasma cortisol is drawn, and at 11 PM dexamethasone 8.0 mg is given orally. At 8 AM the next morning plasma cortisol is measured. Patients with Cushing's disease have a plasma cortisol level below 50% of baseline. Do not confuse this high dose dexamethasone study with the overnight study (1.0 mg dexamethasone) used to screen patients for Cushing's syndrome.

TSH or Thyrotropin

Serum TSH levels are elevated in primary hypothyroidism and are low in hyperthyroidism. If hypothyroidism is suspected on the basis of pituitary disease, then there are usually signs and symptoms to suggest loss of other tropic hormones. Isolated TSH deficiency is a rarity. Pituitary disease is likely when the T4 and T3U values are low and the TSH is "normal." However, patients with pituitary disease seldom have T4 values below 3.0 μg/dL since the thyroid still produces some T4 that is not TSH dependent. Serum T4 values that are very low (<3.0 μg/dL) indicate primary thyroid disease; very low serum T4 and normal TSH suggest binding protein aberration. TRH stimulates a rise in serum prolactin at least three times above basal value. TRH does not raise serum GH levels in normal subjects. In 70–80% of acromegalics, TRH stimulates GH levels to rise (often 10–30 times baseline), a finding that has been as reliable as the use of the oral glucose tolerance test in making the diagnosis of acromegaly. The TRH study has also been used to follow patients receiving therapy for acromegaly to assess how treatment modified the course of their disease.

Follicle-Stimulating Hormone and Luteinizing Hormone

Serum follicle-stimulating hormone (FSH) levels in postpubertal females range between 4 and 15 mIU/mL in the follicular and luteal phases and between 10 and 50 mIU/mL at midcycle. Postmenopausal females, females with primary ovarian failure (e.g., surgical removal, Turner's syndrome), and males with primary hypogonadism have elevated FSH values (40–350 mIU/mL). LH levels in the female again vary with the phase within the menstrual cycle: follicular (4–30 mIU/mL); midcycle (30–150 mIU/mL); and luteal (4–40 mIU/mL). Luteinizing hormone (LH) levels are raised in the postmenopausal female and in the postpubertal patient with primary hypogonadism (>40 mIU/mL). If there is a question of hypopituitarism in a postmenopausal female, one should measure the serum FSH and LH. Finding elevated serum gonadotropins (which are normal and appropriate for the estrogen deficit state) weighs strongly against hypopituitarism. Gonadotropin-releasing hormone (gonadorelin) is available to be used in a few select patients with secondary hypogonadism and in an occasional patient in whom there is a question of whether the pituitary gonadotropes are functioning normally. Gonadotropin-releasing hormone 100 μg iv is given, and blood is drawn at 0, 30, and 60 minutes. LH response to gonadotropin-releasing hormone is greater than FSH and normally rises to values between 25 and 80 mIU/mL by 30 minutes. An intact response excludes gonadotrope dysfunction, but an impaired or absent response cannot be used to define the anatomic abnormality (pituitary vs hypothalamus).

Prolactin

Prolactin is secreted by the pituitary lactotrope. The lactotrope is under tonic inhibition by a hypothalamic substance called prolactin inhibitory factor that is probably dopamine. The upper limit of normal is 20 ng/mL for females and 15 ng/mL for males. The lower limits of detectability in the prolactin RIA do not distinguish between low and normal prolactin levels. Serum prolactin is elevated in many situations. Females with amenorrhea/oligomenorrhea or galactorrhea and males with impotence as well as patients with suspected or known pituitary tumor need to have their serum prolactin measured. Prolactin produces hypogonadism by several mechanisms, leading to low estrogen levels in females and testosterone deficiency in males. Prolactin inhibits the pulsatile secretion of gonadotropin-releasing hormone necessary for the midcycle LH surge and inhibits the positive feedback of estrogen on gonadotropin secretion. Very high levels of prolactin may directly inhibit gonadal function. Prolactin values above 200 ng/mL are seen in two conditions: prolactinoma and chronic renal failure. Prolactinomas (prolactin-secreting pituitary adenomas) may produce prolactin serum levels above 1000 ng/mL. Other causes of hyperprolactinemia include lactation in postpartum mothers, functional hyperprolactinemia (no identifiable pituitary tumor), hypothalamic disorders such as sarcoidosis, histiocytosis, parasellar tumors, and stalk lesions (all presumably decrease prolactin inhibitory factor which releases the lactotrope to secrete prolactin), and pharmacological agents that decrease monoamines or monoamine action (i.e., lower dopamine, the putative prolactin inhibitory factor). These drugs include methyldopa, reserpine, phenothiazines, tricyclic antidepressants, and narcotics. Drugs such as metoclopramide may raise prolactin values as high as 100–150 ng/mL. Patients with primary hypothyroidism (TRH stimulates prolactin secretion) and patients with chest wall diseases and spinal cord lesions (tactile stimulation of nipple areola stimulates prolactin release) may have elevated serum prolactin levels. The prolactin levels in patients with chronic renal failure return to normal after transplantation but not with dialysis.

Dehydration Test

The dehydration study is used in the evaluation of polyuria and polydipsia. Most often the differential diagnosis is among neurogenic diabetes insipidus, nephrogenic diabetes insipidus, or primary polydipsia (psychogenic or compulsive water drinker). Diabetes mellitus is easily excluded by identifying glycosuria and elevated blood sugar. Plasma osmolality (largely determined by the serum sodium concentration) is the primary stimulant of vasopressin release. As plasma osmolality rises, osmoreceptors in the hypothalamus signal adjacent neurons of the supraoptic and paraventricular nuclei to release vasopressin, which is stored in the distal axons of these nuclei terminating in the pituitary stalk and posterior pituitary gland. Vasopressin or antidiuretic hormone (ADH) levels are available in only a few centers, so dehydration is used as the biological assay to assess the action of ADH on the kidney. ADH concentrates urine by increasing the water permeability of the collecting tubules. In the absence of ADH, urine is dilute and its osmolality low.

Normal (ad libitum water) plasma osmolality ranges between 270 and 290 mOsm/kg. If the plasma osmolality and serum sodium are >295 mOsm/kg and >143 mEq/L, respectively, under conditions of ad libitum fluid intake, the diagnosis of primary polydipsia is excluded. The dehydration test must be carefully performed and the patient closely monitored. If the history suggests significant polyuria, then total fluid restriction is begun at 7–8 AM after baseline body weight and urine and plasma osmolality are determined. In cases of less severe polyuria, total fluid restriction may begin earlier (bedtime) after the same baseline variables are measured. A flow sheet is essential to record responses and should have the following headings: body weight, urine specific gravity (a convenient bedside monitor of urine osmolality), urine volume, and urine and plasma osmolality. Body weight and urine values are assessed hourly. When the urine osmolality stabilizes (specific gravity unchanged at the bedside and lab confirmation that the hourly increase in urine osmolality is <30 mOsm/kg for 3 hours), then blood is drawn for plasma osmolality. A plasma value of >288 mOsm/kg assures adequate dehydration. Some patients surreptitiously imbibe water during the study and thus do not concentrate their urine. After urine osmolality stabilizes, administer <u>aqueous vasopressin</u> 5 U subcutaneously, and measure urine and plasma osmolality 1 hour later. If body weight drops to below 3% of the initial weight, then the test is stopped *after* the plasma and urine osmolalities are measured and the response to aqueous vasopressin performed.

In patients with <u>neurogenic diabetes insipidus</u> the urine osmolality rises >150 mOsm/kg after vasopressin is given. Normal subjects and those with nephrogenic diabetes insipidus do not have a rise in urine osmolality in response to vasopressin. Some difficulty in interpreting this test arises in those patients with diabetes insipidus who have residual capacity to secrete ADH under hypertonic conditions of the dehydration test and in compulsive water drinkers who have diluted the concentration gradient in the renal medulla such that even high levels of ADH cannot produce a normally concentrated urine during the short interval of this test. In these circumstances the clinical assessment is important. If there is still doubt regarding the diagnosis, then the plasma from the dehydration test should be assayed for vasopressin. In diabetes insipidus (neurogenic), the plasma vasopressin levels are low, whereas vasopressin levels are appropriately elevated in primary polydipsia.

ADRENAL TESTS

The adrenal glands secrete several hormones: <u>cortisol</u>, <u>aldosterone</u>, and <u>adrenal androgens</u> from the adrenal cortex; <u>epinephrine</u> and <u>norepinephrine</u> from the adrenal medulla. Of these hormones the glucocorticoid, cortisol, is the most important for sustaining life.

Glucocorticoids

The synthesis and secretion of cortisol are regulated by ACTH, with the most frequent pulsations of ACTH coming between 6 and 8 AM. This accounts for the circadian variation of serum cortisol, with the highest levels occurring around 8 AM (15–25 μg/dL) and the lowest levels between 11 PM and 4 AM (<5 μg/dL). The spontaneous rhythm of cortisol release can be altered by psychological stresses (e.g., mental preparation for major surgery, athletic competition, or college examinations) and physical stresses (e.g., severe illness, surgery, trauma, fever, severe dehydration, or hypoglycemia) as well as changing time schedule (e.g., work at night and sleep during the day). A major stress such as cardiac surgery can increase cortisol production six–fold. However, this does not mean the serum cortisol concentration rises 6-fold. Cortisol is a steroid that is insoluble in aqueous solutions and circulates bound to plasma proteins, primarily to cortisol binding globulin (CBG). CBG acts as sump and buffer such that a 6-fold rise in cortisol secretion may be reflected as a 2- or 3-fold rise in serum cortisol. Cortisol is nearly totally (90%) bound to CBG up to concentrations of 25 μg/dL, but as cortisol concentrations rise above this level the binding capacity of CBG is exceeded and the proportion of unbound cortisol or UC rises greatly. For example, when the total serum cortisol is 40 μg/dL, then the concentration of UC is 10 times higher (10 μg/dL) than when the total serum cortisol is 10 μg/dL (1 μg/dL).

The synthesis of CBG is increased by estrogens, oral contraceptives, pregnancy, and hyperthyroidism, leading to elevated levels of CBG and thus raised serum cortisol concentrations. This is important to remember when trying to suppress plasma cortisol with dexamethasone. A woman taking an oral contraceptive may not have a fall in serum cortisol after an overnight dose of dexamethasone. CBG levels can be elevated on a familial basis as well. CBG levels decrease with hypothyroidism, liver disease, nephrotic syndrome, and multiple myeloma. Despite changes in CBG concentrations, the free or unbound cortisol remains normal as long as the pituitary-adrenal axis is normal.

A fraction of the 8–25 mg cortisol normally secreted by the adrenals each day is found in the urine as UC (<100 μg/24 hours). The actual values for normal UC must be established for each laboratory since extraction of urinary corticoids and specificity of the antibody for these corticoids vary. UC is a reliable means of assessing the adrenal glucocorticoid status, especially where the question of hypercortisolism exists. About three of 100 patients with obesity or chronic illness have elevated or false-positive values. Some cortisol assays have antibodies that cross-react with prednisolone, giving false elevated values in UC and serum cortisol determinations in the patient who takes prednisolone or prednisone (metabolized to prednisolone). UC determination is generally preferable to 17-OHCS for several reasons. UC levels correlate well with cortisol production rates. Because UC is measured by RIA, it is not subject to color interference that often occurs in the 17-OHCS assay when patients take drugs. In addition, 17-OHCS measures end-products and intermediates of cortisol metabolism. Normal 17-OHCS levels range between 2.0 and 6.5 mg/g creatinine. UC and urine 17-OHCS determinations are not reliable in renal failure.

Stimulatory studies of cortisol are necessary for patients in whom adrenal insufficiency is suspected. Numerous tests have been used to assess adrenal reserve; the type of study depends on the clinical situation. Often the circumstance may not warrant a provocative study. If the plasma cortisol is elevated ($\geq$18 mg/dL) in a stress situation (e.g., trauma, septicemia, etc.), then stimulatory studies are unnecessary since the pituitary-adrenal axis is intact. If the index of suspicion is low (weak, tired, normally pigmented subject in whom one wishes to exclude Addison's disease), then a short ACTH (cosyntropin) study is ideal (page 11). A normal response (plasma cortisol >18 μg/dL) excludes the diagnosis of primary adrenal insufficiency. Patients who have baseline values of $\geq$18 μg/dL are normal and may not have further rises in plasma cortisol with cosyntropin since they probably are maximally stimulated with endogenous ACTH. Several authors use an increase of >7 μg/dL above 0 time as a normal response. That might be valid in patients with low serum protein (low CBG) in which the plasma cortisol will not reach 18 μg/dL.

If the cortisol fails to increase with the short cosyntropin study, then check concomitant plasma ACTH and cortisol. If the ACTH is significantly elevated and the cortisol is low, then the diagnosis of primary adrenal insufficiency is established. For confusing and confounding data, a formal inpatient study may be necessary to confirm the diagnosis of primary or secondary adrenal insufficiency. **A 24-hour urine is collected as baseline for 17-OHCS and/or UC. Cosyntrosyn, 0.25 mg, in 500 mL saline is infused over 8 hours (8 AM to 4 PM) on 3 consecutive days with concomitant 24-hour urine collections for 17-OHCS and/or UC determinations.** Patients with primary adrenal insufficiency have no rise in the 17-OHCS or UC, whereas patients with secondary adrenal insufficiency have a subnormal rise on the 1st day (less than three times basal 17-OHCS) and increases to three times the baseline by the 3rd day. A shorter method using a 48-hour continuous infusion (cosyntropin 0.25 mg in 500 mL normal saline every 12 hours) is equally valid (normal response: urine 17-OHCS >27 mg in first 24 hours; >47 mg in second 24 hours).

Mineralocorticoids

Excessive mineralocorticoid secretion is suspected in patients with hypertension and hypokalemia. It is important to assess whether the renin-angiotensin system is activated. <u>What is the plasma renin activity?</u> Plasma renin activity can be assayed by eliciting a pressure response in an animal (bioassay) but is most often assayed by RIA measuring angiotensin II. Normal values must be established for each method and laboratory. <u>Plasma renin activity varies with posture, volume status, and sodium content of diet.</u> Plasma renin activity is low, and the aldosterone production is increased in states of mineralocorticoid excess.

Care must be taken to make sure patients suspected of hyperaldosteronism have volume expansion (sodium intake at least 120 mEq/day for 4 days) when measuring urine potassium and aldosterone. Hypokalemia and renal wasting of potassium may resolve with sodium restriction. A urine potassium of >30 mEq/24 hours is inappropriate in the presence of hypokalemia and suggests aldosterone excess. The normal range for urine aldosterone under sodium loading is <20 µg/24 hours. <u>Urine measurements are superior to plasma determinations of aldosterone in making the diagnosis of hyperaldosteronism.</u> However, in differentiating the causes of primary aldosterone excess (adenoma vs hyperplasia), measurement of plasma aldosterone appears to be a better discriminator. Plasma aldosterone, drawn at 8 AM while the patient is recumbent and after being in the supine position overnight, ranges normally between 4 and 12 ng/dL. In patients with an aldosterone-secreting adenoma, plasma levels are >20 ng/dL. Plasma aldosterone levels in patients with bilateral hyperplasia average 13 ng/dL, demonstrating that plasma levels are not helpful in separating these patients from normal individuals.

Adrenal Androgens

The adrenal cortex secretes androgens that have weak masculinizing activity. If concentrations of these weak androgens are high, then some clinical effect is possible (e.g., hirsutism, amenorrhea, voice change, and increased muscle mass in females or prepubertal males). Dehydroepiandrosterone and its conjugated sulfate are secreted in milligram amounts each day and are measured as 17-ketosteroids in the urine. Plasma determinations of dehydroepiandrosterone sulfate can be performed on unextracted serum (normal male and female values; 80–400 µg/dL). Measurement of the serum dehydroepiandrosterone sulfate is more convenient than collecting 24-hour urine for 17-ketosteroids. Measurement of the serum dehydroepiandrosterone sulfate or urine 17-ketosteroids may be helpful in states of masculinization or virilization. In many patients with adrenal carcinoma, urine 17-ketosteroids are higher than urine 17-OHCS.

Adrenal Medulla

The catecholamines, <u>norepinephrine and epinephrine</u>, are made in the adrenal medulla. Catecholamines circulate at very low levels in the plasma, making determinations of plasma catecholamines technically difficult. However, urine concentration of catecholamines can be readily assayed using fluorometric or high-pressure liquid chromatography methods for free norepinephrine (normal, $10–70$ μg/24 hours) and epinephrine (normal, $0–20$ μg/24 hours). <u>The metabolites of catecholamines include metanephrine, normetanephrine, and vanillylmandelic acid.</u> Total metanephrines in the urine are <1.3 mg/24 hours. Urinary vanillylmandelic acid is normally <7 mg/24 hours.

Urine studies are ordered when the clinical suspicion for increased adrenergic discharge is high. Are there symptoms that suggest pheochromocytoma (e.g., headache, excessive perspiration, palpitations, hypertension, neuroma, cafe-au-lait spots, multiple endocrine adenomatosis, and family history)? Which study to order (vanillylmandelic acid, free catecholamines, metanephrines) is difficult to decide. The biochemical determination one uses depends largely on the confidence and the reliability of the laboratory. Vanillylmandelic acid performed using the Pisano method is reliable as are methods that use high-performance liquid chromatography. Drugs such as thiazide diuretics and the α-blockers can be used during the urine collection. No special diet is needed while the urine is collected. Many drugs cause fluorescence (e.g., tetracyclines, ephedrine nasal spray, α-methyldopa), so free catecholamines determined by fluorometric assays might give erroneous values. Urinary total metanephrines are elevated by methyldopa, phenothiazines, and monoamine oxidase inhibitors. Each assay (vanillylmandelic acid, total metanephrines, free catecholamines) detects 90% of the patients with pheochromocytoma. Generally two different studies are helpful in discerning the occasional patient who may have a false-negative study. Serial measurements of urines collected daily may smoke out the rare patient with pheochromocytoma that is not seen with a 1-day collection.

PARATHYROID TESTS

Serum Calcium

Normal values for total serum calcium vary depending on the laboratory and range between 8.5 and 10.2 mg/dL. About half of the total serum calcium binds to protein (albumin), and the other half circulates as unbound or ionized calcium. Any disturbance in the serum albumin affects the value of the total serum calcium; each gram of albumin above or below 4 g/dL changes the serum calcium by about 0.8 mg/dL. For example, a serum calcium of 7.8 mg/dL is normal when the albumin concentration is 3 g/dL ("corrected" calcium, 8.6 mg/dL). Similarly a serum calcium of 11.0 mg/dL is not abnormal if the serum albumin is 5.0 mg/dL. A serum calcium of 10.5 mg/dL is inappropriately high when the serum albumin is 3.0 g/dL ("corrected" calcium, 11.5 mg/dL). Many laboratories measure ionized calcium as well as total serum calcium. The parathyroid glands are the primary moment to moment regulators of the serum calcium. The level of ionized calcium determines whether the parathyroid secretes PTH. A low serum ionized calcium stimulates PTH release. PTH causes bone resorption by indirectly activating osteoclasts and stimulating osteocytic osteolysis; increases renal hydroxylation of 25-hydroxyvitamin D to form 1,25-dihydroxyvitamin D, which stimulates intestinal absorption of calcium; and promotes renal tubular reabsorption of calcium. Each of these actions increases serum calcium that in turn decreases PTH secretion.

Parathyroid Hormone

Intact (1–84)PTH has a short half-life of 2–5 minutes, being rapidly degraded to amino terminal (1–34) peptide and a carboxyl terminal (35–84) peptide. The intact PTH and amino terminal fragment are biologically active. The inactive carboxyl terminal fragment circulates about 10-fold higher concentrations than intact PTH (the amino terminal is virtually undetectable). Previous RIAs for PTH could not detect low levels of PTH and have been replaced by immunometric or "sandwich" assays. Antibodies prepared against different regions of the intact PTH give excellent results in these assays. Still, about 10–15% of patients with surgically proven hyperparathyroidism have PTH levels within the normal range (although inappropriate for the degree of calcemia). PTH decreases renal tubular reabsorption of phosphate, which leads to phosphaturia and increases renal tubular secretion of cyclic AMP. Phosphate excretion measuring the tubular resorption of phosphate/glomerular filtration rate is historically one of the oldest methods to assess PTH action. Measurement of urinary cyclic AMP has also been used to assess PTH action.

Suggested Readings

Frohman LA: Diseases of the anterior pituitary. In Felig P, Baxter JD, Broadus AE, Frohman LA (eds): *Endocrinology and Metabolism,* ed 2. New York, McGraw-Hill, 1986, pp 247–337.

Galen RS, Gambino SR: *Beyond Normality: The Predictive Value and Efficiency of Medical Diagnoses.* New York, John Wiley & Sons, 1975, pp 16–19.

Hawkins JB, Burch WM: Rapid tests of adrenocortical function: intravenous versus intramuscular administration of synthetic ACTH. *N C Med J* 50:306, 1989.

Kao PC, van Heerden JA, Grant CS, et al: Clinical performance of parathyroid hormone immunometric assays. *Mayo Clin Proc* 67:637, 1992.

Liddle GW: Tests of pituitary adrenal suppressibility in the diagnosis of Cushing's syndrome. *J Clin Endocrinol Metab* 12:1539, 1960.

Lindholm J, Kehlet H, Blichert-Toft M, et al: Reliability of the 30-minute ACTH test in assessing hypothalamic-pituitary-adrenal function. *J Clin Endocrinol Metab* 47:272, 1978.

Rose LI, Williams GH, Lauler DP, Jagger PI: The 48-hour adrenocorticotropin infusion test for adrenal insufficiency. *Ann Intern Med* 73:49, 1970.

Utiger RD: The thyroid: physiology, hyperthyroidism, hypothyroidism, and the painful thyroid. In Felig P, Baxter JD, Broadus AE, Frohman LA (eds): *Endocrinology and Metabolism,* ed 2. New York, McGraw-Hill, 1986, pp 389–472.

Chapter 2

Endocrine Emergencies

DIABETIC KETOACIDOSIS

Diabetic ketoacidosis (DKA) is the most common endocrine emergency. Immediate diagnosis and aggressive management with careful attention to detail reduce the mortality of this life-threatening disorder to <2%. Clinical <u>symptoms</u> of uncontrolled diabetic acidosis include excessive thirst and dry mouth, polyuria, weight loss, air-hunger, nausea (often with vomiting), weakness, muscle aches, headache, abdominal pain, and central nervous system depression with drowsiness and stupor that may progress to coma. There are often symptoms related to a coexistent infection. <u>Signs</u> of DKA are dehydration with dry mucous membranes, dry skin with poor turgor, and sunken eyeballs; tachypnea often deep and labored; a characteristic fruity odor to the breath; tachycardia; and hypotension.

Laboratory evidence of DKA includes blood glucose >300 mg/dL, serum bicarbonate <15 mEq/L, arterial blood pH <7.30, and plasma acetone is positive at 1:2 dilution. The nitroprusside reaction (crushed Acetest tablet on which one drop diluted plasma is reacted for 2 minutes) detects acetone and acetoacetate but not β-hydroxybutyrate, the major ketone body in DKA. <u>Undiluted</u> serum may give a strong acetone reaction in states of starvation alone. Serum potassium may be low, normal, or high, but total body potassium is depleted. Serum sodium is usually normal but may appear low if the serum is lipemic. Serum amylase is often elevated, falsely suggesting pancreatitis, but raised amylase levels usually result from acetone that interferes with the assay or from amylase from the salivary glands.

<u>Expediency is most important, so one should not wait for every laboratory result before instituting therapy.</u> Serum electrolytes,

26

plasma glucose, blood urea nitrogen, calcium, phosphorus, magnesium, and complete blood count are obtained. Urine is collected for analysis and culture if indicated. A bladder catheter is not used in an alert patient. A baseline ECG is obtained, and a chest X-ray is usually indicated. Nasogastric suction is necessary for the comatose patient. Management of DKA requires fluid replacement, insulin administration, correction of electrolyte abnormalities, and investigation of precipitating causes. If possible the patient should be treated in an acute care unit where close monitoring is available. Because much of the therapy listed below is administered concomitantly and multiple blood determinations are needed to optimize patient care, a well-planned flow sheet is a necessity.

Fluid Replacement

An intravenous line using at least a 19-gauge needle or catheter is established. The typical adult DKA patient needs 6–10 L to replete the fluid status. Normal saline is administered to the hypotensive patient whereas most patients are given 0.45% saline solution (half normal saline) because the plasma osmolality is already greatly elevated. The infusion rate should be rapid (1000 mL for the first 30 minutes, 1000 mL for next hour, then 300–500 mL/hour over first 24 hours). The rate varies depending on urine output, blood pressure, and the circulatory response to a large volume load. As soon as the blood sugar falls below 250 mg/dL, then dextrose 5% in water is infused.

Insulin Administration

There are many regimens for giving regular insulin. <u>Each works as long as there is intensive hourly monitoring of patient's status and recognition of how prior treatment has worked.</u> The use of bolus intravenous insulin, subcutaneous insulin every 2 hours, intramuscular insulin every hour (provided there is good tissue perfusion), or continuous intravenous drip (with or without a starting bolus) does not matter; **paying close attention to the patient does**. Because hypokalemia and hypoglycemia are less frequent with "low dose" regimens, I prefer to give a bolus of 10 U iv regular insulin followed by a constant infusion of 6 U/hour (up to 12 U/hour if there is infection or 2 U/kg/24 hours). If there is no response in the blood sugar or if the acidemia is not being corrected within 3 hours, then higher insulin doses are used. Regular insulin is *not* stopped when the plasma glucose falls below 250 mg/dL, but dextrose 5% is started and the amount of insulin infused per hour decreased. Intermediate insulin should not be given until the patient is stabilized and able to drink and eat food (see page 56–57 for diabetic orders for the hospitalized patient).

Correct Electrolyte Abnormalities

Because of the acidemia and osmotic diuresis of DKA, a typical patient has lost 600 mEq sodium, 400 mEq potassium, 400 mEq chloride, 400 mEq bicarbonate, and 100 mEq phosphate. If the initial serum potassium is >5.5 mEq/L, then no KCl is added to the initial intravenous fluids. If the serum potassium is normal, then sufficient KCl is added to each liter of fluid so that no more than 40 mEq/hour are infused. If the serum potassium is <3.5 mEq/L, then 40–80 mEq/hour are given with close monitoring of the ECG and serum potassium determinations at least every 2 hours. Both serum potassium and serum phosphorus fall after fluid and insulin are started, and a portion of potassium replacement may be given as potassium phosphate. Any suggestion of renal impairment means less aggressive potassium replacement.

The serum phosphorus may fall below 1.0 mg/dL during therapy. Phosphate deficiency reduces erythrocyte 2,3-diphosphoglycerate levels, thereby increasing hemoglobin affinity for oxygen and decreasing oxygen availability to tissue. Although there has been no difference in the mortality or morbidity rates between patients who have had regimens of phosphorus replacement and those using standard therapy, phosphorus supplementation has been recommended. Patients with hypophosphatemia on admission are at risk to develop severe hypophosphatemia with insulin therapy and are most likely to benefit from phosphorus supplementation. Phosphate may be given at the rate of 10–15 mmol/hour in the form of a buffered potassium phosphate solution (Abbott, 3 mmol phosphorus/mL and 4 mEq potassium/mL), adding 5 mL of this solution to each liter of intravenous fluid. If phosphorus is used, one should measure serum calcium every 4–6 hours since hyperphosphatemia causes hypocalcemia and possible tetany. Addition of phosphate is contraindicated in renal insufficiency.

Use of bicarbonate therapy in DKA is controversial. There are some good reasons to avoid bicarbonate administration. With acute alkalinization, there is a paradoxical fall of cerebral spinal fluid pH leading to central nervous system depression (worsening of stupor/coma) and a shift in the hemoglobin oxygen disassociation curve (Bohr effect) leading to tissue hypoxia. However, if the pH is <7.1 and death seems near, then two ampules of sodium bicarbonate (144 mEq sodium and bicarbonate) should be added to 1 L hypotonic saline 0.45% and infused over 1 hour. Avoid giving bolus bicarbonate. The goal is to raise the pH to 7.2–7.25. Lactate is not used in DKA because some patients, particularly hypotensive subjects, already have elevated blood lactate levels.

Investigate Precipitating Cause

This is necessary since any overt or occult infection can lead to DKA. Complete blood count, urine analysis, chest X-ray, and appropriate cultures should be performed as soon as possible. In addition one should consider whether there is an acute myocardial infarction by ECG. Did the diabetic patient take his or her insulin? Was the patient told what to do in situations where insulin requirements might increase (e.g., infection)? Is the patient hyperthyroid?

Certain risk factors that predispose patients with DKA to higher mortality include delay in making the diagnosis or instituting appropriate therapy, advanced age, deep coma, uremia, and myocardial infarction. <u>One goal of DKA treatment is to educate the patient so that recurrences of DKA can be avoided.</u>

HYPEROSMOLAR COMA

Patients with hyperosmolar nonketotic coma usually have Type II diabetes mellitus. They present after an interval (usually 7–14 days) of prolonged osmotic diuresis leading to dehydration. These patients often do not recognize the seriousness of their illness because there is no nausea, vomiting, and air-hunger induced by ketosis. Progressive mental obtundation and convulsions (often focal seizures) lead to medical consultation. The mortality in these patients approaches 40% mainly because of advanced age, complicating illnesses (hypertension, renal insufficiency, congestive heart failure, stroke), and the presentation for medical care late in the illness. There is often some precipitating factor such as pneumonia, sepsis, urinary tract infection, drug administration (diuretics, glucocorticoids, phenytoin), intravenous hyperalimentation, tube feeding without sufficient free water, or dialysis.

Laboratory findings include severe hyperglycemia (>600 mg/dL), hyperosmolality (>320 mOsm/kg), absence of ketosis, and azotemia (blood urea nitrogen 60–90 mg/dL). Plasma osmolality is calculated using the following formula: 2(Na + K) + glucose/18 + blood urea nitrogen/2.8. Serum sodium may be low as a result of the prolonged hyperglycemia. The correction factor is 1.6 mEq/L sodium for each 100 mg glucose/dL above normal serum glucose levels. Patients with normal or elevated serum sodium still have total body depletion of sodium as well as of potassium, magnesium, and phosphorus. If the bicarbonate is low (<15 mEq/L) in the absence of ketonemia, one should think of lactic acidosis.

The treatment is similar to that for DKA. These patients need large amounts of fluids (up to 10 L) given as normal saline. Monitoring of central venous pressure or pulmonary wedge pressure is often necessary to aid in the management of fluids in patients with renal and cardiac failure. As in DKA, meticulous attention to input and output, measurement of serum electrolytes, insulin therapy, an up-to-date flow sheet, and proper identification of precipitating events are important.

HYPOGLYCEMIC COMA
General Description

Severe hypoglycemia causes mental confusion, bizarre behavior, seizures, coma, and finally death. Hypoglycemia should be considered in any comatose patient in whom a specific diagnosis is not established. Insulin-induced hypoglycemia ("insulin reaction"), a complication of insulin therapy for diabetes mellitus, accounts for most cases of hypoglycemia.

Treatment

Managing hypoglycemic coma requires urgency to prevent brain damage.

1. Obtain blood for plasma glucose determination. Plasma can be stored for insulin measurement if the cause of hypoglycemia is not known.
2. Administer 50 mL of 50% dextrose intravenously over 3–5 minutes. If the patient does not awake during this interval, administer another 50 mL of 50% dextrose. If the patient recovers after dextrose, start dextrose 5% in water until hourly blood sugars reveal

no hypoglycemia. If oral hypoglycemic agents have been ingested, the follow-up interval relates to the type of agent and its
biological half-life which may be prolonged (e.g., the effects of
chlorpropamide may last up to 60 hours).
3. Investigate precipitating factors.

Remember glucose administration for alcohol-induced hypoglycemia can unmask thiamine deficiency producing Wernicke's disease (weakness and paralysis of external ocular recti, nystagmus, various palsies of conjugate gaze; ataxia; deranged mental function).

ACUTE ADRENAL INSUFFICIENCY
General Description

Adrenal crisis is relatively easy to manage; the difficult aspect is to
think of the possibility of adrenal insufficiency. The symptoms are
nonspecific (weakness and fatigue, weight loss, anorexia). Patients
with undiagnosed Addison's disease may present with nausea, vomiting, fever, hypotension, and vascular collapse precipitated by various
stresses including infection, trauma, surgery, drugs, cathartics, ene-
mas, and fasting.

One clinical finding suggesting Addison's disease is cutaneous hyperpigmentation, particularly in the creases of the hand, over the
knuckles, in the axilla, on the gingival mucosa, in the areola of the
breasts, and in the perineum. Scars formed after adrenal insufficiency
develops may be pigmented. Vitiligo is also a clue that signals an autoimmune disorder, the most common cause of adrenal insufficiency.

Patients with pituitary disease are also at risk to develop secondary adrenal insufficiency, but the hyperpigmentation typical of
Addison's disease is absent. Bilateral adrenal hemorrhage leading to
crisis (hypotension, fever, nausea and vomiting, confusion) is a rare
occurrence and is usually found in patients with complicated medical
illnesses, especially in those on anticoagulants. They manifest crisis
symptoms in addition to abdominal, flank, or back pain.
Hyperpigmentation and weight loss are absent.

Common laboratory findings in adrenal crisis include hyponatremia, hyperkalemia, and azotemia; anemia, eosinophilia, lympho-
cytosis, hypoglycemia, and hypercalcemia are less frequent. Plasma
cortisol is low in all circumstances. Plasma ACTH level is high in primary adrenal insufficiency.

Treatment

Management of adrenal crisis requires prompt clinical diagnosis, taking of blood for cortisol and ACTH determinations, fluid replacement to combat dehydration and shock, cortisol administration, and identification and treatment of any precipitating causes. Once the diagnosis is suspected, blood is drawn for plasma cortisol and ACTH determination, and therapy is begun at once. This is an emergency situation, and treatment is life-saving.

A large intravenous line is used to give 1–2 L normal saline-dextrose 5% over the first 2 hours. Hydrocortisone sodium succinate (Solu-Cortef) 100 mg is given iv stat, and 100 mg every 6 hours are administered as continuous intravenous drip over the first 24 hours. Solu-Cortef is reduced to 50 mg iv every 6 hours when conditions stabilize. Mineralocorticoids are not needed because cortisol (hydrocortisone) at these large doses (>150 mg/day) has enough salt retaining activity; 3–5 L saline are given during the first 24 hours.

If the previously drawn plasma cortisol returns low and ACTH levels are available, the workup is considerably simplified because a low cortisol value and elevated ACTH confirm the diagnosis of Addison's disease. If ACTH levels are not available, then a cosyntropin study (page 11) should be performed after the crisis has passed. A confirmed diagnosis means chronic maintenance therapy, education about behavior in stress situations, and wearing of an identification medallion (Medic-Alert) stating the medical diagnosis.

THYROID CRISES

Thyroid storm (decompensated hyperthyroidism) and myxedema coma (decompensated hypothyroidism) are diametrically opposite in physiology yet have three features in common: (a) altered mental status, (b) defective thermoregulation, and (c) some precipitating event. This leads to four clinical axioms. If mental status is normal, then the patient does not have thyroid storm or myxedema coma. If there is no problem with temperature, then thyroid storm or myxedema coma is unlikely (an exception is the hypothyroid patient with infection and normal temperature). If the patient has thyroid storm or myxedema coma, there is always a precipitating factor or event. Finally, successful outcome depends on early diagnosis and managing the precipitating event, so "when in doubt, treat."

Thyroid Storm

General Description

Thyroid storm represents a life-threatening syndrome of decompensated thyrotoxicosis. The chronic thermogenesis of hyperthyroidism leads to augmented peripheral blood flow with shunting of blood to the skin for dissipating body heat. The increased vascular dilatation causes expansion of plasma volume (about 1 L), mild dilutional anemia, widening of pulse pressure, and increased heart rate and cardiac output. Thyroid storm usually develops in an <u>undiagnosed</u> hyperthyroid patient who has a major stress precipitating the following clinical syndrome: a severely ill subject with fever (>101°F), marked anxiety and agitation (delirium, stupor, and coma), anorexia with nausea and vomiting, tachycardia (tachydysrhythmias), abdominal pain, pulmonary edema, or cardiac failure. These occur in the setting of other symptoms and signs of hyperthyroidism. Elderly patients may not demonstrate agitation or goiter but rather show apathy, confusion, cachexia, and atrial fibrillation. The precipitating stress may be a medical illness (e.g., infection, DKA), 131-iodine treatment (1–2 weeks later), or a surgical procedure or trauma (e.g., hip fracture). Thyroid storm used to be a major problem during surgery for toxic goiter, but proper treatment to make the patient euthyroid before surgery has alleviated this concern. Blood should be obtained for complete blood count, free thyroxine, total serum thyroxine (T4)/thyroid hormone binding index, thyroid stimulating hormone, and cortisol. Again, to diagnose thyroid storm one must confirm altered mental status and fever and identify the precipitating event in a patient who is thyrotoxic.

Treatment

The treatment of thyroid crisis requires <u>vigorous management of the underlying illness</u>; <u>supportive measures to decrease body temperature</u>; <u>β-adrenergic blockade</u> of catechol-mimetic signs and symptoms of thyrotoxicosis; <u>inhibition of thyroid hormone synthesis</u>; <u>blockade of thyroid hormone release from the thyroid gland</u>; and <u>inhibition of the conversion of T4 to triiodothyronine (T3)</u>. The most immediate need is to prevent cardiovascular collapse caused by fever, tachycardia, and heart failure. Reducing the cardiac demands is accomplished by peripheral cooling (ice packs, cooling blankets, fans, etc.) and pharmacologic blockade of central nervous system thermoregulatory center (25–50 mg chlorpromazine and 25–50 mg meperidine iv every 4–6 hours). Use just enough of the chlorpromazine/meperidine to prevent shivering. Supportive measures include digoxin for heart failure (the usual dose needs to be increased 1.5- to 2-fold), antipyretics (acetaminophen or corticosteroids but not aspirin because it displaces thyroid hormones from their binding proteins), and intravenous fluids supplemented with B vitamins. In the nauseated or severely agitated patient, propranolol 1 mg should be given as intravenous boluses every 5–10 minutes (no more than 15–20 mg should be given intravenously). Later propranolol (40–80 mg po) can be given every 6 hours. The major effect is β-adrenergic blockade, but propranolol also diminishes the peripheral conversion of T4 to T3. Esmolol, a short acting β-blocker, may be used if intravenous propranolol is not effective or if there is bronchospasm or heart failure. Esmolol given as a loading dose of 250 μg/kg/minute can be titrated from 50 to 500 μg/kg/minute to maintain pulse at 100 beats/minute. Verapamil may also be administered for atrial fibrillation. Propylthiouracil (PTU) 1000 mg should be given orally or be crushed and given via nasogastric tube; thereafter 300 mg PTU is given every 4–6 hours. It takes 10–20 days to reach maximum PTU effect, but the thionamides (PTU and methimazole) are the mainstay therapy for hyperthyroidism. PTU also blocks T4 to T3 conversion. <u>Iodine is the most effective agent for lowering serum T4 acutely.</u> One hour after the loading dose of PTU is given, start iodine therapy. If iodine is given before PTU, it may fuel the synthesis of more T4, possibly worsening the clinical state. For the patient who cannot take oral medications, sodium iodide 1 g is given by intravenous drip over 12 hours every 12 hours to block preformed thyroid hormone release from the thyroid gland. If the patient can tolerate oral medications, then Lugol's solution 10 drops every 8 hours or saturated solution of potassium iodide five drops every 8 hours serves as well as intravenous sodium iodide. Other forms of iodine work as well (e.g., sodium ipodate 1 g every 24–48 hours). The effect of iodine may last only a few weeks, but by then the thionamides should reach peak efficacy. Although there is no evidence of adrenal insufficiency in thyroid storm, high dose glucocorticoids block the conversion of T4 to T3 and lower body temperature. Thus dexamethasone 2 mg iv every 6 hours is recommended for 24–48 hours.

After beginning treatment for thyroid crisis the patient should improve markedly during the first 12 hours even before serum T4 falls.

The patient's temperature, tachycardia, tremor, and mental status should improve during the first day's treatment, but the congestive heart failure may take days to resolve; the atrial fibrillation may take up to 2 weeks to revert to normal rhythm. Muscle weakness may improve during the first few hours after therapy, but strength returns to normal only weeks later.

Myxedema Coma

General Description

The diagnosis of myxedema coma should be considered in every case of stupor or comatose state with hypothermia and in which there is no other obvious cause. Hypoglycemia is another endocrine disorder presenting in a similar manner. Myxedema coma is the rare and very serious (mortality up to 66%) end stage of hypothyroidism. Most often the patient has had unrecognized hypothyroidism for some time, and a precipitating event leads to myxedema coma. Precipitating factors include pulmonary infection, congestive heart failure, general anesthesia and surgery, drugs (sedatives, narcotics, antidepressants), and exposure to cold. An elderly person not known to have hypothyroidism may develop myxedema coma during the winter. A history of previous thyroid hormone therapy, radioactive iodine treatment, a thyroidectomy scar, or goiter are clues to the correct diagnosis. In addition, the patient usually has physical findings of prolonged hypothyroidism (dry skin, puffy eyelids and face, large tongue, hyporeflexia, bradycardia). These patients have marked peripheral vasoconstriction mediated by relatively unopposed α-adrenergic stimulation that result in reduced total blood volume (about 1 L), diastolic hypertension, decreased cardiac output, and reduced heart rate. These patients are cold to touch, reflecting peripheral vasoconstriction.

Respiratory failure is the major cause of death in myxedema coma. The respiratory center becomes insensitive to hypercarbia and hypoxia, creating a vicious cycle of progressive respiratory depression, reduced cardiac output, and increasing cerebral hypoxia. Pulmonary infection often complicates these events. Hypoventilation leads to hypercapnia and respiratory acidosis. Defective hypothalamic thermoregulation causes decreased body temperature (hypothermia). Additional findings include dilutional hyponatremia, anemia, and occasionally hypoglycemia and cortisol deficiency. Blood should be drawn for laboratory testing (complete blood count with differential, free T4 or T4/thyroid hormone binding index, thyroid stimulating hormone, plasma cortisol), but treatment should not be delayed to await the thyroid/cortisol results. White cell count is normally low to normal in hypothyroidism, so a normal white blood cell count with a shift to the left suggests infection.

Treatment

Myxedema coma should be treated in an acute care unit since these patients often require ventilatory assistance. "Intubate early" is a good rule. Drugs that suppress respiration should be avoided. Identifying the precipitating event is imperative (infection, drug overdose, surgery, hypothermia, myocardial infarction). Even though edematous, be judicious with any diuretic since these patients are volume deplete; any slight change in volume could precipitate shock. Any infection is treated vigorously. Hypothermia should be corrected by passive warming with blankets, rather than active warming devices that increase caloric need, induce peripheral vasodilation, and accentuate the hypotension. Avoid inadvertent overdosing with sedatives, tranquilizers, diuretics, and digoxin that can be precipitating factors for myxedema coma. Drugs are cleared slowly, so normal doses of many medications need to be reduced and intervals between doses lengthened. Although the effect of most drugs are potentiated by hypothyroidism, warfarin is a notable exception owing to altered clearance of vitamin K-dependent clotting factors. The blunted effects of warfarin in hypothyroidism are reversed in hyperthyroidism where the effect of warfarin is enhanced.

Thyroid hormone replacement is essential, and most endocrinologists administer L-thyroxine intravenously. This is in contrast to the usual treatment of hypothyroidism where small doses of T4 are titrated over several weeks to reach the euthyroid state. The potential risk of aggressive therapy is accepted in view of the mortality rate in myxedema coma. L-Thyroxine 500 μg is given as intravenous bolus. This dose saturates T4 binding sites that serve as a depot for free T4. Alternatively, one could use L-triiodothyronine 30 μg administered intravenously as a single dose (Triostat) and then 15 μg every 12 hours in addition to oral T4 100–200 μg/day. I also recommend glucocorticoid coverage (Solu-Cortef 100 mg every 6 hours as continuous intravenous drip) until results of the initial plasma cortisol are known. Temperature, pulse, blood pressure, and mental status should improve within 24 hours. Intravenous fluids should be administered carefully. Hyponatremia will be corrected by T4 alone; no saline administration is necessary. A maintenance dose of T4 50–100 μg iv as a single daily bolus is given until oral medications can be taken. At that time L-thyroxine 1.7 μg/kg body weight/day po is prescribed.

HYPERCALCEMIC CRISIS
General Description

The signs and symptoms of severe hypercalcemia are not specific. The patient may have hyperparathyroidism or some other medical illness frequently associated with hypercalcemia (e.g., malignancy). In this setting, an intercurrent disorder such as a viral infection or progression of the underlying disease leads to anorexia, nausea, vomiting, and weakness. The combination of inadequate fluid intake and the inability of hypercalcemic patients to conserve free water leads to volume contraction that raises the total serum calcium level to over 14–15 mg/dL. The degree of calcemia needs to be interpreted in relation to the serum protein concentration since approximately half of the serum calcium is bound to albumin; the other half (ionized or free Ca) is the metabolically active component. In general, for each g/dL of albumin above or below 4 g/dL, the serum calcium can be "adjusted" upward or downward by 0.8 mg/dL. For example, if the serum calcium is 12 mg/dL and the albumin 2 g/dL, then the "corrected" serum is nearly 14 g/dL, which has much more significance. The magnitude of the hypercalcemia correlates well with the severity of the clinical status. Dehydration, confusion, and lethargy are signs that should trigger aggressive management. Untreated severe hypercalcemia leads to coma, muscular paralysis, and ventricular arrhythmia (QT shortening on the ECG).

Treatment

Management of hypercalcemic crisis involves <u>volume repletion and hydration</u>. In normal states of hydration approximately 70% of the filtered calcium load is reabsorbed by the proximal renal tubule, but in states of volume contraction over 90% of the calcium is reabsorbed, accentuating the hypercalcemia. Use a large bore indwelling intravenous needle to deliver 1000 mL normal saline during the 1st hour, realizing that these patients are at least 4–5 L deficient in fluid. Thereafter normal saline is infused at 250–300 mL/hour. Volume repletion often decreases the hypercalcemia to less than critical levels (<13 mg/dL).

If the clinical status is not satisfactory after hydration alone, then the renal excretion of calcium can be enhanced by saline diuresis. The rate of saline administration must be individualized depending on cardiac and renal status. Central venous pressure or pulmonary wedge pressure monitoring is helpful. After hydration is assured, furosemide 40–60 mg every 4–6 hours is given intravenously with careful recording of input and output. Urine volumes losses are replaced with intravenous normal saline. With these measures the serum calcium generally falls 3–4 mg/dL within 24 hours. If renal function does not permit saline diuresis, peritoneal or hemodialysis can reduce the calcium concentration.

Another effective means to lower serum calcium is to decrease bone resorption. Because increased resorption of bone is the etiology of 99% of hypercalcemias, any agent that blocks osteoclastic function will lower the serum calcium. Several hypocalcemic drugs include diphosphonates, plicamycin, calcitonin, and gallium nitrate. These agents work best in the acute situation since their effects are short-lived and tend to be less effective on repeated administration. That is why it is so important to treat the underlying malignancy—the most common cause of the hypercalcemic crisis.

Pamidronate (Aredia), a diphosphonate, reduces the hypercalcemia of malignancy and greatly facilitates its management. After adequate hydration is assured, pamidronate 60–90 mg is given intravenously over 24 hours. By 24 hours, serum calcium levels start to fall. Its effect peaks at 5–6 days and lasts up to 3 weeks. Lower doses are necessary (30 mg) if there is renal insufficiency. Sodium etidronate (Didronel), a diphosphonate, is also safe and effective. Sodium etidronate is administered intravenously in 3 L saline/day at a dose of 7.5 mg/kg/day. Seventy-five percent of patients with cancer achieve normal serum calcium levels after 3 consecutive days of treatment. Longer infusions (up to 7 days) may be necessary. Patients should be well hydrated, so renal function will not be adversely affected. If the serum creatinine >3 mg/dL, use another calcium-lowering agent.

Plicamycin (mithramycin) is an effective medication. At a concentration 1/10 of its therapeutic dose in treating testicular neoplasm, mithramycin inhibits osteoclast differentiation. Within 24 hours after plicamycin (25 μg/kg iv over 8 hours), the serum calcium falls and stays reduced for 7–14 days. The major side effect is thrombocytopenia; plicamycin is both hepatotoxic and nephrotoxic.

<u>Calcitonin</u> also decreases serum calcium but not as well or for as long as plicamycin. The potential side effects of calcitonin are small compared with plicamycin. Salmon calcitonin, 4–8 MRC U/kg sc, is given every 12 hours. Intradermal skin testing should be performed; it is quick and may avoid anaphylaxis that rarely has been reported. The hypocalcemic effect lasts for 48–72 hours, after which tachyphylaxis usually develops.

<u>Gallium nitrate</u> inhibits bone absorption. Gallium nitrate is administered by continuous intravenous infusion at 200 mg/m^2/day for 5 days. It can be nephrotoxic and should not be given with aminoglycosides.

Other medications sometimes lower serum calcium. Glucocorticoids (prednisone 40–60 mg/day) decrease the serum calcium in some malignancies (e.g., lymphoproliferative types), in sarcoidosis, and in vitamins A and D intoxication. Salicylates (600 mg every 6 hours) or indomethacin (75–150 mg/day) inhibit prostaglandin synthetase, which might cause the humoral hypercalcemia of malignancy, but their efficiency is sporadic and unpredictable. Intravenous phosphates work well, but the precipitation of calcium phosphate salts within body tissues has led to their very infrequent use. Oral phosphates (10 mL phosphosoda tid) may be used in some chronic hypercalcemic patients particularly if renal function is normal. Because immobilization tends to exacerbate hypercalcemia, early ambulation is strongly recommended.

In summary, emergent care (calcium >14 mg/dL) requires vigorous saline infusion, saline diuresis, calcitonin injection, and plicamycin since these modalities have most rapid onset of action. Rarely, hemodialysis is required. Then other modalities such as pamidronate are added. Again, treatment of underlying malignant disease is the key for long-term care of the hypercalcemia. If primary hyperparathyroidism caused the hypercalcemic crisis, then surgical intervention is recommended.

HYPOCALCEMIC CRISIS
General Description

Hypocalcemia causes neuromuscular irritability. The severity of neurologic disorder correlates with the degree of hypocalcemia. It is the ionized calcium level that is the crucial factor rather than the total serum calcium. In the absence of any serum protein abnormalities or any acid-base derangements, the total serum calcium is quite reliable in assessing the calcemic status. In acute hyperventilation, the total serum calcium is normal, but the ionized calcium is low due to increased protein binding of calcium in alkaline conditions. Hypoalbuminemia of chronic disease leads to hypocalcemia but not to any clinical hypocalcemic syndrome since the ionized calcium is normal. Acidosis raises serum ionized calcium levels.

Hypocalcemic crisis presents as overt tetany: carpopedal spasm, spasm of the laryngeal muscles with stridor, muscle cramps, and occasionally seizure. Chronic hypocalcemia sometimes presents with papilledema related to benign intracranial hypertension. Cardiac arrhythmias are seen with the typical ECG finding of a prolonged QT interval caused by ST lengthening. The cause of the hypocalcemia may be obvious: operative parathyroid damage related to thyroid or parathyroid surgery; multiple blood transfusions (citrate complexes calcium and, if not metabolized by the liver, leads to hypocalcemia); acute pancreatitis; or rickets and osteomalacia. Hypocalcemia caused by idiopathic hypoparathyroidism, vitamin D deficiency (e.g., gastrointestinal disease with malabsorption), or hypomagnesemia may not be so obvious. Hypomagnesemic hypocalcemia is frequent in chronic alcoholics and is occasionally found in patients with intestinal malabsorption syndromes. Whenever the total body magnesium is low (serum magnesium <1.2 mg/dL), parathyroid hormone synthesis and release are inhibited, leading to hypocalcemia. Correction of the hypomagnesemia restores normocalcemia.

Hypocalcemic tetany must be distinguished from the muscle spasms that result from *Clostridium tetani* infection of a wound. The spasms of tetanus begin in the head and neck (trismus), whereas the spasms of tetany occur in the extremities (carpopedal spasm). Strychnine poisoning presents with clonic spasms, not tetanic spasms. Seizures in infants caused by hypocalcemia may be aggravated by usual treatment with anticonvulsants. Phenytoin and phenobarbital decrease serum vitamin D levels, leading to less calcium absorption by the intestine.

Emergency laboratory assessment consists of immediate serum calcium and ECG to assess the QT interval. Serum levels for magnesium, phosphorus, total protein/albumin, blood urea nitrogen, electrolytes, and parathyroid hormone are obtained before therapy.

Treatment

Hypocalcemic crisis is treated by intravenous infusion of calcium. Concentrated calcium is very irritating to the veins, so dilute two 10-mL ampules of 10% calcium gluconate into 100 mL of 5% dextrose and infuse over 10–15 minutes. This may be repeated every 4–6 hours for recurrence of symptoms. Although the serum calcium falls quickly to pretreatment levels after the intravenous bolus, hypocalcemic symptoms and signs may not return for several hours. Alternatively, a constant infusion of 15 mg calcium/kg every 4–6 hours may be given. Calcium gluconate 10% has 9 mg elemental calcium/mL of solution. Monitoring the serum calcium level is important. If hypomagnesemia is found, then magnesium sulfate 1 g im (8.13 mEq or 98 mg elemental magnesium) given three times daily for 3–5 days replaces body reserves and corrects the hypocalcemia. For patients taking intravenous fluids, an intravenous drip of magnesium sulfate (98–196 mg every 8 hours for 3–5 days) can be used to avoid painful intramuscular injections. For transfusion hypocalcemia, 10 mL of 10% calcium chloride should be given for every 2 U citrated blood. Finally, those patients with chronic hypocalcemia (page 170) who require calcium supplementation and vitamin D replacement must wear proper identification concerning their medical diagnosis (e.g., Medic-Alert).

Patients who have diabetes mellitus, diabetes insipidus, adrenal insufficiency, and hypoparathyroidism and those receiving chronic glucocorticoids should carry a card or preferably a bracelet or medallion listing diagnosis, medications, and attending physician. Lack of such information could prove disastrous in emergency situations when the patient is not conscious. Bracelets and medallions are available from the following nonprofit organization: Medic-Alert Foundation International, 1000 North Palm Street, PO Box 1009, Turlock, CA 95380.

Suggested Readings

Axelrod L: Diabetic ketoacidosis. *Endocrinologist* 2:375, 1992.

Benua RS, Becker DV: Thyroid storm. In Bardin CW (ed): *Current Therapy in Endocrinology & Metabolism*, ed 4. Philadelphia, Decker, 1991, pp 68–70.

Fisher JN, Shahshahani MN, Kitabchi AE: Diabetic ketoacidosis: low dose insulin therapy by various routes. *N Engl J Med* 297:238, 1977.

Foster DW: Insulin deficiency and hyperosmolar coma. *Adv Intern Med* 19:159, 1974.

Foster DW, McGarry JD: The metabolic derangements and treatment of diabetic ketoacidosis. *N Engl J Med* 309:159, 1983.

Gaich G, Burtis WJ: The diagnosis and treatment of malignancy-associated hypercalcemia. *Endocrinologist* 1:317, 1991.

Nicoloff JT: Thyroid storm and myxedema coma. *Med Clin North Am* 69:1005, 1986.

Rapoport B: Myxedema coma. In Bardin CW (ed): *Current Therapy in Endocrinology & Metabolism*, ed 4. Philadelphia, Decker, 1991, pp 79–82.

Schade DS, Eaton RP, Alberti KGMM, Johnston DG: *Diabetic Coma: Ketoacidotic and Hyperosmolar.* Albuquerque, University of New Mexico Press, 1981.

Singer FR, Fernandez M: Therapy of hypercalcemia of malignancy. *Am J Med* 82(suppl 2A):34, 1987.

Chapter 3

Diabetes Mellitus

Diabetes mellitus is the most common endocrine disorder encountered in medical practice. The complications of this chronic disorder of glucose homeostasis are a major cause of disability and morbidity.

DIAGNOSIS OF DIABETES MELLITUS

Diabetes mellitus is easily diagnosed when there is unequivocal elevation of the plasma glucose (>200 mg/dL) with classical symptoms of polyuria, polydipsia, polyphagia, and weight loss. However, some patients may not have this degree of hyperglycemia or these symptoms. In these patients an <u>oral glucose tolerance test</u> (GTT) is used to establish the diagnosis of diabetes mellitus. The National Diabetes Study Group has made recommendations for the standardization of testing and has established criteria for the diagnosis of diabetes mellitus that are very useful. By these criteria, diabetes mellitus is present when **(*a*) <u>fasting plasma glucose is >140 mg/dL on two occasions or (*b*) fasting plasma glucose is <140 mg/dL and 2-hour plasma glucose is >200 mg/dL with one intervening value of >200 mg/dL after a 75-g glucose load (GTT).</u>**

Normal glucose values of nonpregnant adults are fasting plasma glucose <115 mg/dL and 2-hour plasma glucose <140 mg/dL. Older tests give criteria for whole blood, but most glucose determinations are now performed on plasma with results that average 15% higher than whole blood glucose. The GTT should be performed only on subjects who have been on an unrestricted diet containing at least 300 g carbohydrate/day and who have been physically active for 3 days before the test. A 75-g glucose load should be administered in the morning after a 10-hour fast. The patient should remain seated and should not smoke during the study. Blood is drawn at 0, 30, 60, 90, and 120 minutes.

GTT is not recommended in the following circumstances: (*a*) when fasting hyperglycemia is already present; (*b*) in hospitalized patients or acutely ill patients or patients who are physically inactive (e.g., bedridden); or (*c*) subjects taking medications such as diuretics, propranolol, phenytoin, glucocorticoids, estrogens, and birth control pills.

Some patients have impaired glucose tolerance (fasting plasma glucose <140 mg/dL; 2-hour plasma glucose >140 mg/dL (but <200 mg/dL); and an intervening value >200 mg/dL) after the 75-g load. These subjects have an abnormality in glucose metabolism intermediate between normal and overt diabetes. It may worsen to diabetes, improve toward normal, or remain unchanged on serial testing. It is best to label these patients impaired glucose tolerance rather than diabetes mellitus.

GTTs on pregnant women are interpreted somewhat differently. The criteria for gestational diabetes mellitus are those of O'Sullivan. Diabetes mellitus is diagnosed during GTT when there are two or more plasma glucose concentrations that meet or exceed the following criteria: fasting, 105 mg/dL; 1-hour, 190 mg/dL; 2-hour, 165 mg/dL; 3-hour, 145 mg/dL. Pregnant females normally have fasting glucose levels 10–30 mg/dL below the subject's nonpregnant fasting value.

CLASSIFICATION OF DIABETES MELLITUS
Diabetes Mellitus Type I

These patients are insulin deficient because of islet β-cell loss and require insulin replacement therapy. Type I diabetes mellitus usually has its onset in youth. These patients are prone to ketosis and often present in diabetic ketoacidosis. Type I diabetes is frequently associated with specific human leukocyte antigen types that may predispose to viral insulitis or autoimmune phenomena (e.g., islet cell antibodies). The inheritance is complex and not simple Mendelian. The family history is more likely negative for diabetes mellitus Type I. Even if an identical twin develops Type I diabetes mellitus, the other twin has only a 50% chance of developing diabetes.

Diabetes Mellitus Type II

This is the common form of diabetes affecting nine of ten patients with diabetes. Typically these patients are overweight adults (at least 80% are obese). The diabetes relates to a combination of defects.

Tissue insensitivity to circulating insulin (insulin resistance) is nearly universal, leading to hepatic overproduction and tissue underutilization of glucose. The plasma insulin levels are often elevated but are less than expected in normal subjects given the same degree of hyperglycemia, and there is a delay in insulin secretion after glucose challenge. The family history is usually positive and often shows the pattern of autosomal dominant inheritance. Type II patients generally do not develop ketosis because they have enough insulin to inhibit lipolysis. As the duration of diabetes increases, many patients fail to produce enough insulin even while taking oral hypoglycemic agents. These patients need supplemental insulin, making them insulin-requiring Type II diabetics. A small subset of Type II patients develops diabetes at an early age (maturity-onset diabetes of youth (MODY)). Table 3.1 indicates the differences between Type I and Type II diabetes mellitus. Categorizing patients to either type helps to think about pathophysiology, but not all patients fit neatly into such typing (e.g., thin, geriatric diabetics and those Type II patients who fail with oral hypoglycemics often require insulin treatment).

Secondary Diabetes Mellitus

This form of diabetes results from loss of pancreatic tissue owing to pancreatitis or surgery or from hormone antagonism to insulin action as in acromegaly and Cushing's syndrome.

Impaired glucose tolerance designates glucose tolerance results intermediate between normal and overt diabetes. This has been discussed in relation to the GTT. The basis of this separate classification rather than including it in Type II diabetes is the observation that the development of overt diabetes in such patients occurs at a rate of

Table 3.1
Classification of Diabetes Mellitus

Diabetes Mellitus	Type I	Type II
Age of onset (yr)	<40 (often <20)	>40
Family history	Rare	Common (95%)
Ketosis prone	Yes	No
Specific human leukocyte antigen associations	Yes	No
Obesity	Rare	Common (80%)
Insulin sensitivity	Sensitive	Resistant
Requires insulin	Yes	Generally not

1–5%/year. Such an impairment of glucose tolerance may not be associated with long-term microangiopathic and neuropathic complications of diabetes mellitus.

Lipotrophic diabetes mellitus is a rare hyperglycemic syndrome characterized by severe insulin resistance, partial or total absence of body fat, high circulating levels of insulin, absence of ketosis, and hepatomegaly that often progresses to cirrhosis.

COMPLICATIONS OF DIABETES MELLITUS

The long-term complications of diabetes mellitus are the same regardless of classification (Type I, Type II, or secondary diabetes). Chronic hyperglycemia leads to hyperlipidemia, hypercholesterolemia, and glycosylation of proteins that are presumed to cause microvascular and atherosclerotic changes. However, the development of the following complications is heterogeneous and unpredictable in any one patient with diabetes. What distinguishes the diabetic patient who lives 40 years with no to minimal problems from the nearly blind, azotemic patient with 20 years of diabetes is not well understood. Control of blood glucose is one factor, but the innate capacity to "heal and repair" may be just as important.

Diabetic Retinopathy

Background (nonproliferative) retinopathy is characterized histologically by focal dilatations of capillary walls (microaneurysms) and clinically by "dot" or "blot" hemorrhages, soft gray-white exudates (representing microinfarction of superficial nerve fibers), and retinal edema. Although microaneurysms cannot be seen with the ophthalmoscope, intraretinal hemorrhages (dot or blot hemorrhages) can be detected with the ophthalmoscope. Background retinopathy increases with the duration of the disease such that half of the patients with diabetes mellitus for 10 years manifest this form of retinopathy. It usually does not cause any visual impairment unless retinal edema, plaques of hard exudates, or hemorrhage occur in the macula itself. Macular edema represents further progression of retinopathy. The macula, the central portion of the retina critical for color vision and fine acuity, suffers in diabetes with edema from capillary damage. Unfortunately, macular edema cannot be appreciated by direct ophthalmoscopy; only a trained observer using stereoscopic viewing through a slit-lamp biomicroscope can detect the characteristic retinal thickening.

Proliferative retinopathy represents further progression, and its presence signifies an ominous state. Diabetes is the leading cause of blindness in the United States mainly due to proliferative retinopathy. New vessels, containing no mural pericytes to support their endothelium, are very fragile. These new vessels proliferate in response to ischemia and are often located at the disc margins. Because of their fragility, these vessels are subject to hemorrhage into the retina and vitreous. Finding proliferative retinopathy has great clinical importance. The incidence of severe visual loss increases from 1.5%/year to nearly 20%/year after proliferative retinopathy is first identified. Fluorescein angiography is helpful in evaluating retinopathy because it identifies severe intraretinal hemorrhage and early neovascularization. Treatment consists of photocoagulation to decrease oxygen requirements throughout the retina and thus retard the neovascular process. In cases of persistent vitreous hemorrhage that have not cleared over 1 year, surgical removal of the vitreous (vitrectomy) has been relatively successful in restoring useful vision. Because early detection of proliferative retinopathy and appropriate treatment save vision, patients who have had diabetes more than 10 years should schedule annual visits with the ophthalmologist.

Diabetic Nephropathy

About 30–35% of Type I patients develop end-stage renal disease that requires either dialysis or renal transplantation for survival. End-stage renal disease is more prevalent in Type I diabetes than Type II and three times more common in blacks than in whites. Hyperfiltration and increased creatinine clearance occur early in diabetes. Later, microvascular changes in the kidney, including thickening of the basement membrane and mesangium of the glomerulus, are associated with increased glomerular permeability resulting in proteinuria. Normally, albumin content in a 24-hour urine collection is <15 mg. Microalbuminuria, defined as 24-hour urine containing ≥30 mg albumin but less than 300 mg, heralds the onset of diabetic renal disease. Best results come from quantitative determinations on 24-hour collections. The traditional dipstick registers positive only after albumin excretion exceeds 10 times the normal rate. Typically, microalbuminuria is not present in the first 5–10 years of Type I diabetes. Hypertension, a less sensitive marker of diabetic renal involvement, correlates well with the degree of albuminuria and the duration of diabetes. Proteinuria of 3–5 g/day usually leads to hypoalbuminemia and edema (nephrotic syndrome). Persistent proteinuria (>300 mg/day) is an ominous sign because renal failure usually develops within 5 years after its appearance. Once azotemia is present, progressive development to frank uremia occurs within 3–4 years.

Management of patients with diabetic nephropathy requires controlling glycemia, normalizing blood pressure, correcting hyperlipidemia, and slowing the progression of proteinuria. Urinary tract infections are common in diabetics and need to be treated appropriately. Aggressive treatment of any hypertension appears to stall end-stage renal disease. Angiotensin-converting enzyme inhibitors (captopril, enalapril, lisinopril) are most effective and do not adversely affect the lipid status. Cough (up to 10% of angiotensin-converting enzyme-treated patients) and allergic congestion of nasal mucosa (3% of patients) may limit their use. Treating patients with microalbuminuria with angiotensin-converting enzyme inhibitors appears to delay renal disease. Calcium channel blockers have been used, but the verapamil-type blocker causes bradycardia and may trigger congestive heart failure by reducing cardiac output. Peripheral α-1 blockers (prazosin, terazosin) also help by maintaining renal perfusion without affecting lipid levels. Diuretics have side effects that worsen hyperglycemia, elevate triglycerides, and deplete stores of sodium, potassium, and magnesium. Nevertheless, reduction of fluid retention achieved by diuretics means that these agents are unavoidable in managing manifestations of advancing nephropathy. Treatment of diabetic renal failure is difficult. Medicare in the United States makes the question of dialysis nearly moot. Criteria for institution of hemodialysis or renal transplantation have to be formulated in view of each center's experience since these patients do not fare as well as those with nondiabetic renal failure.

Diabetic Neuropathy

Up to 50% of patients with longstanding diabetes develop a neurologic problem. Diabetic neuropathy is one of the earliest clinically detectable complications of diabetes mellitus. Of the several forms of diabetic neuropathy, <u>peripheral neuropathy</u> (symmetrical segmental demyelination of long nerve axons) is most common and is manifested by loss of ankle deep tendon reflexes and decreased vibratory sensation in the lower extremities. Patients complain of an insidious onset of numbness, tingling, and a burning sensation that is characteristically worse at night. Ultimately, there is a glove-and-stocking loss of pin prick and light touch sensation. Neurotrophic ulcers may develop in areas of repeated trauma (such as that caused by poorly fitting shoes or unattended calluses). Loss of pain perception may lead to neurotropic arthropathy (Charcot's joints), which is typically located in the tarsal-metatarsal area bilaterally.

Mononeuropathy is a disorder of a single nerve or nerve root (typically the femoral, sciatic, lateral femoral cutaneous, or third cranial nerves) thought to be due to infarction following occlusion of a vasa nervorum. Pain in the distribution of the affected nerve is the most troublesome symptom. The diabetic third nerve palsy (ptosis, ophthalmoplegia) can be differentiated from a more ominous intracranial process (aneurysm, cavernous sinus thrombosis) by preservation of the pupillary response to light in the diabetic-related mononeuropathy. A unilateral bandlike thoracic or abdominal pain (radiculopathy) may initially mimic herpes zoster or a thoracic or abdominal emergency. Mononeuropathy usually has a good prognosis, with spontaneous return of function and resolution of pain within 3–18 months.

Diabetic amyotrophy leads to weakness of the pelvic girdle muscles or, less commonly, the shoulder muscles. There is no associated pain. Diabetic amyotrophy is best seen in the hands with wasting of the interosseous muscles, particularly over the dorsum next to the second metacarpal bone (first dorsal interosseous muscle).

Autonomic neuropathy produces postural hypotension, impotence, retrograde ejaculation, hypotonic bladder, gastroparesis, and diabetic diarrhea. Loss of vagal tone to the heart leads to diminished sinus arrhythmia (loss of R-R variability) and later sinus tachycardia. Sudomotor changes produce distal anhidrosis and troublesome central hyperhidrosis (increased facial and truncal perspiration). Diabetic neuropathic edema results from increased blood flow and pronounced vasodilatation with arteriovenous shunting caused by sympathetic denervation. Autonomic neuropathy can lead to hypoglycemia unawareness, a troublesome and potentially lethal complication of insulin administration, in which counter-regulatory responses to hypoglycemia are impaired.

Management of polyneuropathy is directed to symptomatic relief of pain with non-narcotic analgesics, exquisite foot care (toe nails trimmed, avoidance of hot water soaks, properly fitting shoes, gentle abrasion of corns and calluses with a pumice stone). Better control of diabetes may improve the neurological symptoms. Treatment with medications is still very empirical; many have been tried, and each regimen has had its proponents. Such medications include amitripty-line (50–100 mg at bedtime often prescribed with fluphenazine 1 mg, if no effect in 6 weeks then discontinue), phenytoin (100 mg tid, if no effect in 2 weeks then discontinue), carbamazepine (starting with 200 mg/day increasing up to 800 mg/day, if no effect at 800 mg/day then discontinue), antihistamines (diphenhydramine 50 mg tid), and vitamin preparations such as Brewer's yeast tablets (three tablets qid). All have met with varying success. Patients with amyopathy respond best to insulin treatment rather than oral hypoglycemic agents.

Atherosclerotic Cardiovascular Disease

Arteriosclerosis is accelerated in diabetes mellitus; as a result, coronary artery disease and peripheral vascular disease are significant causes of morbidity and mortality. The postmortem incidence of coronary artery occlusion is five times more frequent in diabetics than in nondiabetics in all decades of life and regardless of sex. The immediate mortality rate of acute myocardial infarction is similar to the nondiabetic population (30–55%), but the long-term prognosis in the diabetic is quite different, with a 5-year survival of 38–43% compared with 49–83% in nondiabetics. Diabetic females are as likely to have myocardial infarction as diabetic males.

Peripheral artery occlusion is a common complication leading to claudication, rest pain, ulcer formation, and gangrene. Peripheral arterial disease is often associated with diabetic neuropathy and local infection, leading to the diabetic foot (see "The Diabetic Foot"). Five of every six major leg amputations for ischemic disease of the foot occur in patients with diabetes mellitus. As a general rule, arteriosclerosis in diabetes mellitus has an increased incidence, occurs at an earlier age, is more rapidly progressive and accentuated, and carries a more severe prognosis than in nondiabetics.

The combination of neuropathy, arterial vascular disease, hyperglycemia ± ketoacidosis sets up for certain life-threatening infections that are nearly unique for diabetes. Soft tissue and fasciae involvement of the lower extremities (infected diabetic foot, necrotizing cellulitis, necrotizing fasciitis, clostridial myonecrosis (gas gangrene)), external auditory canal (malignant external otitis), and sinuses (rhinocerebral mucormycosis) require prompt surgical debridement and antimicrobial therapy. Another common infection in diabetes is candidiasis. Hyperglycemia helps *Candida* infections by glycosylating the active site on complement (C3), so opsonization of bacteria is inhibited, and by inducing protein synthesis in *Candida*, similar to the polymorphonuclear leukocyte complement receptor, so that normal leukocyte-complement interaction will be interrupted.

MANAGEMENT OF DIABETES MELLITUS

Probably nowhere else in medical therapeutics are there more ways to manage a problem than in diabetes mellitus. The ideal management of diabetes would lead to a normal lifestyle; normal glucose, fat, and protein metabolism; avoidance of hypoglycemia; prevention of long-term complications; and satisfactory psychosocial adaptation to living with a chronic disease. These goals can be achieved in acute diabetes (diabetic ketoacidosis, hyperosmolar coma) but are usually only transiently achieved in the daily care of patients with diabetes mellitus. Seventy years of experience with insulin therapy have not prevented the long-term complications of this disorder. Although 20% of patients with diabetes mellitus never develop complications, there is no way in advance to detect these "protected" patients. Much laboratory data suggest that achievement of euglycemia is the best way to prevent these complications. The most comprehensive clinical study, Diabetes Control and Complications Trial (DCCT), showed that intensive insulin therapy (three to five injections per day or insulin pump, four to seven finger stick glucoses per day, and weekly checks with diabetic team) vs conventional insulin therapy (two injections per day) reduced diabetic complications in patients with Type I diabetes. The DCCT found that intensive treatment decreased retinopathy by 76%, reduced the progression of existing retinopathy by 51%, decreased the need for laser therapy by 50%, lowered the rate of early renal disease by 42% and more severe disease by 51%, and prevented neuropathy by 60%. The best insurance to avoid long-term complications of diabetes is to maintain the blood sugar as close to normal as possible. If the physician is lackadaisical, this attitude is transferred to the patient and reflects how he or she will handle his or her diabetes.

The most crucial time to share the philosophy of management as well as the specifics about how to achieve these goals is immediately after the diagnosis is made (first office visit, first hospitalization). It is very difficult to change habits once they are established. The time to initiate regular diet, weight control, insulin dosage, and so forth is not when the patient finally presents with symptomatic neuropathy, claudication, or loss of vision. To prevent these complications requires a committed approach early in the disease. Patient education is the primary factor in achieving adequate control. A team approach that uses the expertise of a dietitian, diabetic teaching nurse, and physician is ideal.

Diet and Weight Control

A well-balanced diet eaten regularly at breakfast, lunch, and dinner (bedtime snack for those patients receiving insulin) is necessary. A diet composed of 50% carbohydrate, 20% protein, and 30% fat is reasonable, but food preferences and socioeconomic situations should be used to determine the precise regimen. Consultation with the dietitian is quite helpful.

The number of Calories (kcal) recommended is based on body weight and activity. Ideal body weight (IBW) for adult females with a medium frame approximates 100 lb plus 5 lb for each inch over 5 feet. Thus, a 5'2'' woman's IBW is 110 lb. For a small frame, deduct 10% from IBW; for large frame, add 10% of IBW. For medium frame males, the IBW is 106 lb plus 5 lb for each inch over 5 feet. Subtract or add 10% of IBW for a small or large frame, respectively. Thus, a 6'1'' large frame man's IBW would be 188 lb [106 + (5 × 13)] + 10% [106 + (5 × 13)].

The total Calorie requirement each day is the sum of the basal requirements plus the activity requirements. Basal Calorie requirement is IBW times a factor of 10 (IBW × 10). The Calorie requirements based on activity follow: sedentary lifestyle, IBW × 3; moderate activity, IBW × 5; heavy work activity, IBW × 10. Thus, a 5'10'' medium frame construction worker would require 1560 Cal (IBW × 10) + 1560 Cal (assume heavy work activity (156 × 10)) for a total of 3120 Cal each day to maintain body weight. A less complicated formula that calculates the number of Calories needed to maintain body weight is body weight (lb) × 12.

When patients need weight reduction, decreasing total Calorie intake to 500 Cal/day less than maintenance will produce a 1-lb weight loss each week (1000 Cal/day will give a 2-lb weight reduction each week). All patients need repeated dietary instructions to reinforce dietary habits.

Diabetic Control

Control is difficult to define. Ideal control mimics the plasma glucose variation in normal subjects. The level of hyperglycemia must be arbitrarily set for each patient and his or her particular circumstances. For example, the degree of hyperglycemia permitted is greater for a

75-year subject than for an otherwise healthy 23-year individual mainly because of the risks of hypoglycemia (insulin reaction) in the elderly. In general, a preprandial blood glucose level of <140 mg/dL represents acceptable control. <u>Strong motivation and good education make the difference between good and poor diabetic control.</u> There are two advances in diabetic care that bear on control: glycohemoglobin determinations and self-monitoring of blood glucose.

Glycosylated Hemoglobin

Nonenzymatic addition of glucose to proteins occurs in the body and in the test tube. High glucose concentrations favor the formation of these stable glycoproteins. When the hemoglobin A is glycosylated, hemoglobin A1c is formed. Normally, hemoglobin A1c represents <6% of the total hemoglobin (range varies with different assay techniques). Technically, it is easier to measure glycosylated hemoglobin as hemoglobin A1 (normal values are <8%). In poorly controlled diabetics, hemoglobin A1c accounts for >10% of the total hemoglobin. Glycosylated hemoglobin correlates with the degree of glycemia during the last 6–8 weeks (half-life of erythrocytes is about 120 days) and gives an integrated value (in contrast to blood sugar which fluctuates widely). When properly performed, the glycosylated hemoglobin helps to confirm whether the control of blood sugar has been "on the average" what the patient says it has been. Remember any states of hemolysis cause falsely low glycosylated hemoglobin levels. Whether glycosylation of proteins in general has any direct role in the pathogenesis of diabetic complications (micro- or macrovascular disease) is uncertain.

Self-Monitoring of Blood Glucose

Patients are active participants in the care of their diabetes. They are responsible for insulin injections and for testing and recording their blood glucose or urine sugar before meals and at bedtime. <u>Monitoring these variables is the only way to assess whether the insulin regimen is controlling the diabetes.</u> Home monitoring of blood glucose (Dextrostix, Chemstrip bG, etc.) is especially helpful in planning therapy. Finger puncture with disposable lancets using an automatic, spring-loaded apparatus (Autolet, Autoclick, etc.) facilitates blood sampling and is practically painless. The reagent strips for checking the blood glucose are reliable when care is taken to follow directions, but they cost $50–60/100 strips. When starting insulin, getting blood sugar levels before meals and at bedtime provides a rational basis for insulin recommendations. Later, particularly for the patient with sore fingertips (prick the side of the fingertip—it is less sensitive) or few funds or for better compliance, ask for one reading a day, but stagger the times. Obtain and record before breakfast blood glucose one day, before lunch the next, before dinner the next, then at bedtime the next and repeat the cycle each day. This allows the patient and you to see if there are patterns of hyperglycemia and/or hypoglycemia. If patients use the information for feedback on diet and insulin administration, then they are more likely to diligently check the blood sugar. If they or you do not use the data, then there is no reason to do finger sticks. If the patient cannot afford this method of monitoring the diabetes, then urine is checked before meals and at bedtime on a "double-void" specimen (empty bladder first, then urinate 15–30 minutes later and check this specimen) using either tablets (Clinitest two-drop method) or reagent strips. The goal for control for those who do not monitor blood sugar is aglycosuria with very infrequent insulin reactions.

Because we can quantitate biochemical parameters, they are most often used as indexes of control. Table 3.2 lists biochemical criteria useful in assessing diabetic control.

Insulin Treatment

The Type I diabetic patient requires insulin to lower blood glucose. If there is some "reserve" of insulin secretory activity from the pancreatic β-cells, then blood sugar is more easily regulated. The amount and type of insulin required vary and depend on dietary intake, activity, and whether there is any residual endogenous insulin production. The normal pancreatic β-cell secretes about half of its output as boluses in response to food; the other half as a continuous output day and night (basal secretion). Insulin therapy in Type I patients uses these patterns to supplement and/or replace insulin. Knowledge of insulin prepara-

Table 3.2
Biochemical Criteria to Assess Control

Descriptive	Fasting Blood Sugar	2-Hour Postcibal Blood Glucose	Hemoglobin A1c	Serum Cholesterol
Excellent (great)	65–115	<140	<6	<200
Acceptable (good)	<140	<200	<7	<200
Fair (not good)	<200	<230	<8	>240
Poor (bad)	>200	>230	>8	>240

tions and their duration of action is necessary. Human regular insulin is rapid acting and when administered subcutaneously begins to have effects 30–45 minutes later, peaks at 2–3 hours, and lasts up 4–5 hours. There are two intermediate acting insulins: neutral protamine Hagedorn (NPH) and zinc suspension (lente) insulin. Each when administered subcutaneously begins to have effects 2–3 hours later, peaks at 4–6 hours, and lasts 8–12 hours. Human NPH action often lasts less time than beef/pork NPH (8 hours vs 12–14 hours, respectively). Figure 3.1 demonstrates a <u>split-mixed</u> program using the combination of NPH and regular insulin taken twice daily. This <u>conventional program</u> offers the advantage of providing insulin throughout the 24-hour day, the convenience of taking only two injections per day, and considerable flexibility in controlling hyperglycemia without producing hypoglycemia. At least 60% of patients taking human NPH before dinner have fasting hyperglycemia necessitating moving the NPH later to bedtime (9–10 PM). This means three injections a day (NPH/regular before breakfast, regular before dinner, and NPH at bedtime).

<u>Insulin regimens need to be individualized.</u> The patient's desire for control, willingness to cooperate, ability to comprehend, resources to monitor blood sugar, lifestyle (age, activity, work schedule), and partial or total need for supplementation enter the equation. For ex-

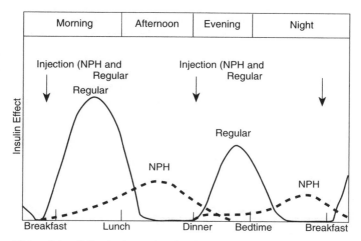

Figure 3.1. Split-mixed program of twice daily insulin. Regular and intermediate insulin are taken together as one injection 30–60 minutes before breakfast and evening meal.

ample, the newly diagnosed Type I diabetic may require total supplementation for few weeks, then only partial for a few months ("honeymoon" phase), then total supplementation. The insulin-requiring Type II often does well with supplements for basal secretion (e.g., NPH twice a day). For some patients who have visual and dexterity problems, premixed insulins (e.g., 70/30—70% NPH and 30% regular) offer convenience. Patients with Type I diabetes are generally started on an intermediate-acting insulin (NPH, lente, or Monotard) ± regular or short-acting insulin. Human insulin is given to patients with newly diagnosed diabetes. This may be done as an outpatient when the patient has only modest symptoms, but many patients will already be hospitalized after presenting with ketoacidosis.

The total insulin requirement (TIR) per day depends on whether there are concomitant problems such as infection or ketoacidosis. To start, figure TIR as 0.6 U/kg/day for a nonstressed adult. An empirical regimen worked out in many insulin-requiring diabetics uses 4/9 of TIR as NPH before breakfast and 1/6 of TIR given as NPH at bedtime. Regular insulin is administered subcutaneously 2/9 of TIR before breakfast and 1/6 TIR before dinner. For physicians who have used a split-mixed twice daily regimen (Fig. 3.1), the dosage is equivalent to giving 2/3 total daily dose in the morning (2/3 as NPH and 1/3 as regular) and 1/3 total before the evening meal (half as NPH and half as regular). Table 3.3 outlines typical orders for managing patients admitted for treatment of diabetes. Table 3.3 is detailed enough to allow changes in insulin dose "to fine tune" the blood glucose.

Table 3.3
Orders for Diabetes Care in a Hospitalized Patient

1. BG (finger stick) must be measured and recorded eight times daily: ac, 1 hr pc, hs, and 3 AM

2. Diet is 25 kcal/kg/24 hr: 50% is carbohydrate, 20% protein, 30% fat

3. TIR for first 24 hr is calculated as 0.6 × body weight (kg) = ___ U; use human insulin unless ordered otherwise

4. NPH insulin orders: 4/9 of TIR before breakfast and 1/6 of TIR at bedtime

5. Regular insulin orders: 2/9 of TIR before breakfast and 1/6 of TIR before dinner

6. 7:30 AM: breakfast NPH = 4/9 TIR = ___ U to be adjusted by the following scale

Table 3.3. *Continued*

Check last predinner BG:
If predinner BG is <70, then decrease morning NPH by 2 U
If predinner BG is 71–120, then no change in morning NPH
If predinner BG is >121, then increase morning NPH by 2 U

Regular = 2/9 TIR = ___ U to be adjusted by the following scale
    BG <70, then give 2/9 TIR − 3% TIR = ___ U
    BG 71–100, then give 2/9 TIR = ___ U
    BG 101–140, then give 2/9 TIR + 3% TIR = ___ U
    BG >141, then give 2/9 TIR + 6% TIR = ___ U
If BG 1hr pc is <110, then decrease corresponding next day mealtime
    regular insulin by 2 U
If BG 1 hr pc is 111–150, then no change in corresponding next day
    mealtime regular insulin
If BG 1 hr pc is >151, then increase corresponding next day mealtime
    regular insulin by 2 U

7. 11:30 AM: prelunch: regular insulin is given based on the following
    scale
    BG <120 = no insulin
    BG 121–140, then give 1/18 TIR − ___ U
    BG 141–180, then give 1/18 TIR + 2 U = ___ U
    BG >181, then give 1/18 TIR + 4 U = ___ U

8. 5 PM: predinner: regular insulin is 1/6 TIR = ___ to be adjusted by the
    following scale
    BG <70, then give 1/6 TIR − 3% TIR = ___ U
    BG 71–100, then give 1/6 TIR = ___ U
    BG 101–140, then give 1/6 TIR + 3% TIR = ___ U
    BG >141, then give 1/6 TIR + 6% TIR = ___ U
    If BG 1 hr pc is <110, then decrease corresponding next day mealtime
        regular insulin by 2 U
    If BG 1 hr pc is 111–150, then no change in corresponding next day
        mealtime regular insulin
    If BG 1 hr pc is >151, then increase corresponding next day mealtime
        regular insulin by 2 U

9. 10 PM bedtime NPH: give 1/6 TIR = ___ U and adjust by the following
    scale
    If ac breakfast BG is <70, then decrease hs NPH by 2 U
    If ac breakfast BG is 71–120, then no change in hs NPH
    If ac breakfast BG is >121, then check last hs and 3 AM BG
    If last hs and 3 AM BG are >121, then increase hs NPH by 2 U
    If 3 AM BG is <70 regardless of hs or ac breakfast BG, decrease hs
        NPH by 2 U
    If hs and 3 AM BG are 70–120, but ac breakfast >121, then increase
        hs NPH by 2 U

BG, blood glucose.

Having a preprinted sheet with these orders simplifies procedures. TIR increases to 0.7 U/kg for a viral syndrome, to 1.0 U/kg for bacterial infection, and to 2.0 U/kg for sepsis, ketoacidosis, or stress doses of steroids.

Three clinical axioms are significant for diabetic control: "provide around-the-clock insulin," "fix the fasting first," and "poor control begets poor control; good control begets good control."

The concept of providing "around the clock insulin" is important for control. Some patients with residual endogenous insulin may need only one injection of intermediate-acting insulin a day. For most patients with diabetes, one injection of an intermediate-acting insulin does not control the blood sugar throughout the day. Increasing the dose to >60 U/day as a single injection greatly increases the risk of hypoglycemia. To avoid these problems and provide around-the-clock basal insulin, split the insulin into two injections of intermediate insulin (before breakfast; before the evening meal or at bedtime) and add a short-acting insulin (regular, Semilente, or Actrapid) if blood sugars at lunch and at bedtime are increased. Another means to cover the 24-hour day is to prescribe human Ultralente insulin at supper (which has a prolonged period of action) as one daily dose and add regular insulin at supper and at breakfast to cover the postprandial state.

Another concept is "to fix the fasting first." If the blood sugars are >150 mg/dL before breakfast, several possibilities should be considered. First, ask if there is evidence of nocturnal hypoglycemia (awake with headache, wet bedclothes, "bad" dreams, or obvious insulin reaction)? If there is evidence of hypoglycemia, then the morning hyperglycemia (or glycosuria) probably reflects the counter-regulatory response to prior hypoglycemia (Somogyi phenomenon). If there is no evidence of hypoglycemia, then assume that the morning NPH is not covering the last 8 hours of the 24-hour clock. An abrupt increase in fasting levels of plasma glucose occurring between 5 and 9 AM without antecedent hypoglycemia is called the <u>dawn phenomenon</u>. The dawn phenomenon is common in insulin-dependent (Type I) and noninsulin dependent (Type II) diabetes mellitus. The best way to correct this is to give beef/pork NPH 30–60 minutes before the evening meal or human NPH at bedtime. Start with 1/6 of TIR (again TIR = 0.6 U/kg/day) and add more if the hyperglycemia persists. Nocturnal reactions are likely to occur when large single doses of NPH are given or when the NPH before the evening meal is excessive. As before, the patient is responsible for monitoring and recording his or her glucose values. In cases where there is persistent hyper-glycemia before bedtime, regular insulin (1/6 of TIR) is administered before the evening meal, which covers that meal and reduces the bed-time hyperglycemia. Both insulins can be drawn up in one syringe and given as a single injection (first drawing up regular and then the NPH to avoid contamination of regular with NPH). Likewise for blood glu-coses levels that are elevated before lunch, regular is added to the morning NPH injection. Whenever there is hypoglycemia (insulin re-actions or blood glucose <60 mg/dL), reduce the dose of the appro-priate insulin. If the individual is a jogger or bicyclist, then insulin should be injected into the deltoid or abdominal areas rather than the thigh to avoid rapid absorption of the insulin and possible hypo-glycemia. The most predictable and less erratic site is the abdomen. If there is a question of absorption, stay with injections in the abdomen (rotating so as not to inject same site within a couple of weeks).

Another concept that relates to control is "poor control begets poor control; good control begets good control." Patients who are chronically hyperglycemic need more insulin to get better glucose control. That is, insulin sensitivity is reduced, requiring greater insulin supplementation than might be needed if they had lower blood glu-coses. A good example is the resistance during and after DKA. Likewise, good control improves insulin sensitivity, meaning less in-sulin in needed.

The DCCT study compared Type I patients receiving conven-tional insulin therapy (usually twice a day split/mixed) with intensive insulin treatment (four injections a day usually regular before meals and NPH at bedtime or insulin pump). Insulin pumps are becoming a practical (although expensive) mode of giving insulin over the entire 24-hour period as well as of giving boluses of insulin before meals. Patient selection for the "pump" requires discernment. These patients must be strongly motivated and dedicated to near normoglycemia. The best pump candidates are those who are those who have wide swings in blood glucose from hypoglycemia to severe hyperglycemia in the same day.

Education is an important facet of long-term diabetic manage-ment. Written instructions to the patient and family are essential. Handouts containing recommendations for diabetic management and algorithms are very helpful in allowing patients to adjust their own in-sulin program and thereby to become responsible for their own dia-betes care on a daily basis.

Complications of Insulin Treatment

Complications that relate directly to insulin administration include hypoglycemia, insulin-induced lipodystrophy, insulin resistance, and insulin allergy.

Hypoglycemia is the most frequent complication of insulin treatment. Recurrent hypoglycemia may be due to (a) omission or delay of meals, (b) unusual heavy exercise, (c) chronic insulin overdosage, or (d) errors in insulin administration or technique. These problems are identified by careful history taking and observation of injection technique and are minimized by patient education. The Somogyi phenomenon (hypoglycemia followed by rebound hyperglycemia) should be suspected in patients who have urine glucoses that vary from negative to strongly positive with ketones within the same 24-hour day and in patients who gain weight despite heavy glycosuria. Monitoring the blood sugar frequently over 24 hours is the best way to confirm this problem.

The immediate treatment of hypoglycemia is with oral carbohydrate (4–8 oz sweetened drink). If the patient is unconscious, administer glucose (50 mL 50% dextrose iv) or glucagon (1 mg im). Dextrose 50% is painful when given intravenously and should be reserved for the unconscious patient. If glucagon is used and the patient does not respond within 15 minutes, administer dextrose 50% because it is unlikely that a second dose of glucagon will be effective.

Lipodystrophy relates to atrophy or hypertrophy of fat at the site of insulin injection. Lipoatrophy is the most frequent and is common in young females. The reaction is due to immune complex formation with less purified insulins and is seen less frequently since the introduction of purer insulin preparations. Lipoatrophy usually resolves within 6–9 months after changing to highly purified insulin that is injected into the periphery of the atrophied area. Repeated injections into the same area cause lipohypertrophy ("insulin tumors"). Frequent rotation of injection sites avoids this problem.

Insulin resistance, defined as a daily insulin requirement of more than 200 U for several days in the absence of ketoacidosis, infection, pregnancy, or an associated endocrinopathy (e.g., acromegaly, Cushing's syndrome, hyperthyroidism), can be divided into three categories: (a) immunogenic insulin resistance (the most common), (b) insulin receptor abnormalities (rare), and (c) local degradation of insulin (rare).

(a) Immunogenic insulin resistance is associated with high titers of anti-insulin immunoglobulin G antibodies to beef insulin and less often to pork insulin. Substitution to human insulin often proves effective. If this does not work, a 2- to 3-week course of glucocorticoids (prednisone 60–80 mg/day) may be tried. Because this regimen may increase resistance to insulin, worsen the hyperglycemia, and has complications inherent to high-dose glucocorticoids, it is best to demonstrate high titers of anti-insulin antibodies before instituting steroids (i.e., prove immunologic insulin resistance) and then manage the patient initially as an inpatient.

(*b*) Insulin receptor abnormalities are associated with acanthosis nigricans (velvety, hyperpigmented areas of skin usually seen around the neck, in the axilla, and in the groin). Anti-insulin antibodies are not present. Two clinical syndromes related to a receptor abnormality are recognized: Type A and Type B. Type A (reduced number of insulin receptors) affects younger females with signs of virilization and accelerated growth related to ovarian androgen overproduction. Type B (antibodies to insulin receptor) affects older women with other signs of immunologic disease such as arthritis, leucopenia, and antinuclear antibodies.

(*c*) Insulin resistance caused by the local degradation of subcutaneously administered insulin and normal sensitivity to intravenous insulin is easily diagnosed by a trial of low-dose intravenous insulin.

Insulin allergy presents usually as a local skin reaction and rarely as a systemic reaction. Local reactions are manifested as induration, erythema, and pruritus at the injection site within 30 minutes to 4 hours of insulin administration and are most likely to occur in patients who have recently started insulin therapy. They relate to an immunoglobulin G-mediated response and resolve spontaneously in most patients after several weeks of continuous insulin therapy. A localized reaction with formation of subcutaneous nodules may be due to preservative (phenol) or zinc within the insulin preparation. Systemic insulin reactions are manifested by generalized pruritus and urticaria, angioedema, or acute anaphylaxis. Systemic reactions can be anticipated by the worsening of local reactions and are most likely to occur in patients who have had prior exposure to insulin but discontinued it temporarily. Treatment with desensitization as an inpatient with appropriate preparation to handle life-threatening anaphylaxis is mandatory. Desensitization is facilitated by a kit available from Eli Lilly, Indianapolis, IN.

Management of Type II Diabetes

Insulin

The very nature of the defect (insulin resistance and altered insulin secretory dynamics) in Type II diabetes usually means that insulin sup-

plementation is not the answer to hyperglycemia. The emphasis in
Type II diabetes mellitus should be on <u>diet and weight loss</u> as primary
therapy. Prescribing insulin to obese patients often leads to a vicious
circle in which insulin lowers blood glucose, stimulates appetite, and
promotes weight gain, leading to more insulin resistance and finally a
return to hyperglycemia. One clear indication for insulin treatment in
Type II diabetes is to cover the acute stress situations such as surgery,
infection, myocardial infarction, and so forth. Many patients with
Type II diabetes require insulin after years of diabetes to control the
blood glucose (β-cell has reached a "state of exhaustion").

Oral Hypoglycemic Agents

Sulfonylurea drugs stimulate insulin release and are used to treat the
hyperglycemia in Type II diabetes, but again <u>use of these hypoglycemic agents in the noncompliant obese subject is usually doomed
to fail</u>. Up to 60% of patients have an initial good response of blood
glucose to these medications, but the sulfonylureas produce effective
long-term results in only 20–30% of patients. There are several sulfonylureas from which to choose. Table 3.4 lists some frequently prescribed agents. Metformin, a biguanide used extensively in Canada
and in Europe, is not available in the United States.

Factors that favor success with sulfonylurea therapy in Type II diabetes include <u>onset of diabetes after age 40</u>, <u>normal body weight or
obesity</u>, <u>known duration of diabetes for <5 years</u>, and <u>no history of insulin therapy</u>. Patients who are underweight are likely to be insulin dependent and usually have a high primary failure rate to sulfonylureas.
Obese Type II patients who still have symptomatic hyperglycemia

Table 3.4
Oral Hypoglycemic Medications

Agent	Daily Dose (mg)	Average Dose (mg)	Cost/Day[a] (¢)
Tolazamide	125–250 bid	500	40
Tolubutamide	500–1000 bid	1500	50
Chlorpropamide	100–500 every day	250	11
Glyburide	2.5–20 every day[b]	7.5[c]	65
Glipizide	5–40 every day[b]	10	60

[a]Cost at average daily dose when generic 100 tablets purchased.
[b]May be given bid.
[c]Micronized glyburide dose 3 mg/day.

(polyuria, fasting blood glucose >250 mg/dL) after 5–10 lb weight loss with diet usually require oral hypoglycemic agents.

The second generation agents, glyburide and glipizide, have less protein interaction so are preferable with patients who take multiple drugs; they however are no more effective as hypoglycemic agents than tolazamide and chlorpropamide. One must be aware that chlorpropamide's prolonged duration of action (24–60 hours) increases the risk of hypoglycemia. Chlorpropamide also may augment the release of vasopressin, leading to hyponatremia and possible water intoxication.

If diet, weight reduction, and oral agents fail to control diabetes, then insulin administration is generally necessary. Several years after the onset of Type II diabetes, many patients lose the ability to secrete insulin and become insulin dependent as well as insulin resistant. These patients require insulin.

Exercise

Exercise is important in weight control and in modulating insulin dosage in diabetes mellitus. Exercise itself has a glucose-lowering effect. However, in the ketotic and severely hyperglycemic patient, exercise will worsen the hyperglycemia. Obese patients especially are encouraged to walk 3–5 miles/day to aid in weight reduction.

THE DIABETIC FOOT

If there is one area that is neglected in diabetic care, it is the feet. Commonsense recommendations and close attention to foot care save limbs and avoid morbidity. The diabetic foot represents the complications of peripheral vascular disease and neuropathy that make the foot and leg susceptible to trivial trauma, skin abrasion, callus formation, and development of ulcers that heal poorly. Often infection intervenes. <u>Always examine the feet of the diabetic patient; make sure that shoes and socks are removed.</u> To miss such an opportunity robs the patient of proper care.

Vascular disease manifests as cold feet, absent pulses, blanching on elevation, dependent rubor, prolonged venous filling time, atrophy of subcutaneous fatty tissues, shiny skin, absent hair on foot and toes, thickening nails, infection, and gangrene. Patients often complain of intermittent claudication and rest pain.

The neurological abnormalities in the diabetic foot lead to the following findings: dry skin, painless traumas, atrophy of intrinsic foot muscles, and fragmentation of bones of the feet (Charcot's joints). Dry skin results from loss of perspiration because of autonomic dysfunction. The dry skin often cracks and fissures, leading to potential sites of infection. Painless trauma caused by loss of sensory nerves is a major problem. Any injury may prove significant: wearing improperly fitting shoes, burns from hot water bottles and heating pads, or trauma from foreign objects such as tacks, nails, and pebbles. Atrophy of intrinsic foot muscles leads to muscle weakness, causing a change in foot shape, gait, and greater pressure on skin areas prone to breakdown (e.g., hammer and claw deformity of the toes puts much more weight on metatarsal heads). Charcot's joint deformity causes increased pressure over bony prominences, leading to ulcer formation.

Prevention is the key to managing the diabetic foot. Table 3.5 provides a means of educating the patient and family about proper foot care. Although simple, adhering to these dos and don'ts means much in terms of hospital dollars, morbidity, and mortality.

SURGERY AND THE DIABETIC PATIENT

Goals for managing the patient before, during, and after a surgical procedure should be clearly identified. These goals include the following. (*a*) Good preoperative control. Control of diabetes makes elective surgery and anesthesia management much easier. Uncontrolled diabetes coupled with the stress of surgery may progress to ketoacidosis or hyperosmolar coma. (*b*) Keep the patient from having hyperglycemia (plasma glucoses >200 mg/dL), which impairs wound healing and increases susceptibility to infection. (*c*) Avoid hypoglycemia.

There are several methods to cover the diabetic patient who needs general surgery. It is important, regardless of the regimen used, that the patient's blood sugars be monitored frequently. Finger stick blood glucose, recorded at the bedside, is rapid and convenient. The frequency of blood glucose checks must be individualized. Most patients are kept fasting after midnight before surgery. An intravenous 5% dextrose solution, 100–150 mL/hour, is started around dawn, and regular insulin is given subcutaneously. The amount and route of insulin administration depend on the patient's normal total daily insulin dose and the type of surgery. The total daily dose is divided by 4. This value is given as regular insulin subcutaneously every 6 hours as long as intravenous fluids are being infused. The first dose is usually given at 7–8 AM on the day of surgery. This regimen is used for all surgery except those operations requiring hypothermia (e.g., car-

Table 3.5
Dos and Don'ts of Diabetic Foot Care

Do

Inspect feet daily for blisters, cuts, and abrasions: if you cannot see the soles, use a mirror; if your vision is poor, get someone to check your feet

Wash feet daily with lukewarm water and soap; dry carefully, especially between toes

Apply hand cream or lanolin to dry areas of feet; be careful not to leave cream between toes

Wear clean socks or stockings daily

Cut nails straight across and file down edges with an emery board

Carefully use a pumice stone or emery board to buff down any dry calluses

Wear well-fitting shoes that do not rub: make sure shoes are comfortable before you purchase them; a wide toebox gives the toes room

Inspect insides of your shoes daily for foreign objects, tacks, or torn linings

Make sure your physician checks your feet at each visit

Don't

Smoke

Wash feet in hot or cold water (check water with elbow to make sure it is lukewarm; a thermometer is even better (85–95°F))

Use a heating pad, heating lamp, or hot water bottle to warm your feet

Perform bathroom surgery (razor blades, scissors) on corns and calluses; leave that for your physician or podiatrist

Use over-the-counter medications on calluses or corns; they can cause chemical burns

Cross your legs when sitting

Wear garters or girdles

Go barefoot; this is especially true on beaches and around swimming pools

Wear shoes without socks or stockings

Wear sandals with thongs between the toes

Wear mended socks or stockings with seams

diac), where absorption may be erratic. In these special situations, regular insulin is given as a continuous intravenous drip at 1–2 U/hour. The rate is increased or decreased according to finger stick blood glucose levels. Blood sugars between 100–200 mg/dL are acceptable.

Postoperatively, a better regimen than the "sliding scale" is to maintain the every-6-hour insulin program and supplement the doses with additional regular insulin in amounts based on the plasma glucose. Additional regular insulin is added to the every-6-hour insulin regimen by using an algorithm based on the blood sugar just before the scheduled injection (the advantage of finger sticks and reflectometer readings at bedside is obvious). For blood sugars between 200 and 249 mg/dL, add 2–4 U; for blood sugars between 250 and 299 mg/dL, add 3–6 U; and for blood sugars >300 mg/dL, add 5–10 U. Using the rule of 5% of the total daily dose for each 50 mg/dL above 200 mg/dL for supplements is helpful. Double the supplements for moderate or large ketosis (unless the ketosis is due to starvation when the plasma glucose levels are reasonable). The exact extra amount varies depending on the basal dose, with the larger amounts being used for patients receiving larger basal doses. If the basal amount needs constant supplementation, then the basal dose is raised; if the blood sugar is low (<60 mg/dL), then the basal dose is reduced. <u>Insulin orders generally require rewriting once or twice daily.</u>

As soon as the patient can eat, regular insulin is given before meals and before bedtime with a bedtime snack. The same dose of regular insulin should not be given before meals and at bedtime because of the overlap of insulin effect with the breakfast dose at 8 AM and the lunch dose at 12 PM and so on. Once the patient can eat, administer the total daily dose of regular insulin as follows: 1/3 before breakfast, 1/6 before lunch, 1/3 before supper, and 1/6 at bedtime. No more than 10 U are given at bedtime, and supplements are not added to the bedtime dose to avoid nocturnal hypoglycemia. Alternatively, the preoperative program may be reinstituted and regular insulin added for anteprandial blood sugars above 200 mg/dL. <u>The importance of monitoring the sugar and making daily adjustments cannot be overemphasized.</u>

The following orders are written as an <u>example to manage</u> the diabetes of a patient who was well-controlled with one dose of 40 U NPH each morning and who was admitted for elective abdominal surgery. They do not take into account other parameters such as electrolyte checks and pre- and postoperative medications.

1. For surgery in morning, nothing by mouth after midnight.
2. Dextrose 5% in water at 125 mL/hour iv to begin at 6 AM.
3. Discontinue current insulin orders.
4. Begin regular insulin U-100 <u>10 U sc every 6 hours at 7 AM</u> (basal regimen).
5. Check blood glucose by reflectometer every 6 hours while on ward (begin at 6:30 AM) and hourly while in operating room and recovery room. <u>Record sugars on flow sheet.</u>
6. Add regular insulin supplements to the basal regimen (10 U every 6 hours) *if* blood sugars are >200 mg/dL. For values 200–249

mg/dL, add 2 U regular insulin; for values 250–299 mg/dL, add 4 U regular insulin; for values 300–400 mg/dL, add 6 U regular insulin; for values >400 mg/dL, call house officer.

7. Postoperatively, continue four times daily regular insulin as long as intravenous lines are running.

8. Nothing by mouth until nausea passes. Begin clear liquids and progress to regular diabetic diet as patient tolerates. Bring tray at 7 AM, 12 PM, 6 PM, and 11 PM.

9. Continue four times daily blood glucose checks and supplemental insulin program.

10. When able to eat home diet program, discontinue intravenous feedings and supplemental bedtime (11 AM) insulin program.

11. Return to home program of 40 U NPH every morning 30–45 minutes before breakfast. Give regular insulin 10 U along with 40 U NPH on the 1st day when starting NPH (will need regular insulin to carry over to 1st day of NPH after being on four times daily regular schedule). Add supplements if needed before meals only (not at bedtime).

12. Make sure nutritionist or dietitian sees the patient to make recommendations.

Suggested Readings

Bagdade JD, Segreti J: The infectious emergencies of diabetes. *Endocrinologist* 1:155, 1991.

Bolli GB, Gerich JE: The "dawn phenomenon"—a common occurrence in both non-insulin-dependent and insulin-dependent diabetes. *N Engl J Med* 310:746, 1984.

Carroll PB, Eastman RC: Insulin resistance: diagnosis and treatment. *Endocrinologist* 1:89, 1991.

Diabetes Control and Complications Trial Research Group: The effect of intensive treatment of diabetes on the development and progression of long-term complications in insulin-dependent diabetes mellitus. *N Engl J Med* 329:977, 1993.

Gavin LA: A comprehensive approach to sidestep diabetic foot problems. *Endocrinologist* 3:191, 1993.

George K, Alberti MM, Gill GV, et al: Insulin delivery during surgery in the diabetic patient. *Diabetes Care* 5(suppl 1):65, 1982.

Gerich JE: Oral hypoglycemic agents. *N Engl J Med* 321:1231, 1989.

Gleckman RA, Roth RM: Diabetic foot infections—prevention and treatment. *West J Med* 142:263, 1985.

Holman RR, Turner RC: A practical guide to basal and prandial insulin therapy. *Diabetic Med* 2:45, 1985.

Mahnensmith RL: Diabetic nephropathy: a comprehensive approach. *Hosp Pract* 28:129, 1993.

McMurry JR Jr: Wound healing with diabetes mellitus: better glucose control for better wound healing in diabetes. *Surg Clin North Am* 64:769, 1984.

National Diabetes Data Group: Classification and diagnosis of diabetes mellitus and other categories of glucose intolerance. *Diabetes* 28:1039, 1979.

Podolsky S: Management of diabetes in the surgical patient. *Med Clin North Am* 66:1361, 1982.

Proietto J: Treatment options in type II diabetes. *Endocrinologist* 2:107, 1992.

Reddi AS, Camerini-Davalos RA: Diabetic nephropathy: an update. *Arch Intern Med* 150:31, 1990.

Shafir E, Bergman M, Felig P: The endocrine pancreas: diabetes mellitus. In Felig P, Baxter JD, Broadus AE, Frohman LA (eds): *Endocrinology and Metabolism,* ed 2. New York, McGraw-Hill, 1986, pp 1043–1178.

Skyler JS, Skyler DL, Seigler DE, et al: Algorithms for the adjustment of insulin dosage by patients who moniter blood glucose. *Diabetes Care* 4:311, 1981.

Watts NB, Spanheimer RG, DiGirolamo M, et al: Prediction of glucose response to weight loss in patients with non-insulin-dependent diabetes mellitus. *Arch Intern Med* 150:803, 1990.

Wender RC: Meticulous glucose control in diabetic persons using insulin. *Compr Ther* 14:16, 1988.

Yudkin JS, Alberti KGM, Mclarty DG, Swai AB: Impaired glucose tolerance: is it a risk factor or a diagnostic ragbag? *Br Med J* 301:397, 1990.

Chapter 4

Hypoglycemia

GENERAL DESCRIPTION

Hypoglycemia must be defined operationally as a blood glucose low enough to produce <u>homeostatic (adrenergic)</u> and/or <u>neuroglycopenic symptoms</u>. <u>Homeostatic symptoms</u> relate to the sympathomimetic stimulation of hormones, including epinephrine, norepinephrine, glucagon, cortisol, and growth hormone, that raise blood glucose in response to hypoglycemia. These homeostatic responses produce the most striking symptoms, including sweating, palpitations, hunger, tachycardia, tremor, and anxiety, and form the early warning signs of hypoglycemia, whereas most neuroglycopenic symptoms occur when the hypoglycemia is more profound. <u>Neuroglycopenia</u> presents as inability to concentrate, confusion, incoherent speech, headache, blurred vision, bizarre behavior, focal or generalized seizures, stupor, coma, and finally death.

A diagnosis of hypoglycemia is made when the patient has the symptoms listed above <u>and</u> plasma glucose levels below 60 mg/dL after overnight fast in both males and females or below 50 mg/dL on an oral glucose tolerance test (GTT) or below 45 mg/dL for females and below 55 mg/dL for males after a 72-hour fast. <u>Symptoms alone do not make a diagnosis of hypoglycemia</u> because most of these reflect a nonspecific increase in adrenergic discharge, nor do low plasma glucose levels alone establish the diagnosis of hypoglycemia unless there are accompanying homeostatic or neuroglycopenic symptoms.

Two other characteristics of hypoglycemic symptoms are their <u>episodic nature</u> and their <u>relief with glucose ingestion</u>. Each episode of hypoglycemic symptoms lasts for minutes up to 1 hour because either counter-regulatory responses spontaneously raise the plasma glucose or the patient eats food to raise the plasma glucose. However, relief of symptoms with food or beverage does not make a diagnosis of hypoglycemia since this is not specific for hypoglycemia.

Several factors (gender, antecedent level of glucose, and rapidity of fall) determine whether a particular level of glucose produces symptoms. Healthy females have a plasma glucose level 10–15 mg/dL lower than males during a 72-hour fast. The antecedent level of plasma glucose is also important because diabetic patients with chronic hyperglycemia may manifest hypoglycemic symptoms at plasma glucose levels of 90–100 mg/dL, whereas normal subjects with glucose levels raised acutely to 300 mg/dL and then reduced abruptly do not have any symptoms until the plasma glucose is reduced to <50 mg/dL. Rapidity of the plasma glucose fall may determine whether symptoms occur, but again the level of glucose itself is the most critical parameter.

CLASSIFICATION OF HYPOGLYCEMIA

Clinically, hypoglycemia can be grouped into three major categories: induced, fasting, and postprandial hypoglycemia.

Induced Hypoglycemia

Induced or exogenous hypoglycemia is caused by the administration of medication (insulin, sulfonylureas, pentamidine, or, rarely, salicylates or sulfonamides) or ingestion of toxic chemicals (alcohol). Induced hypoglycemia is by far the most common cause of hypoglycemia. **Simply stated, the differential diagnosis for any hypoglycemia is (a) medication/drug, (b) medication/drug, (c) medication/drug, and (d) other.** Induced hypoglycemias do not require an exhausting workup, but a carefully taken history is mandatory. For the diabetic with insulin reactions, the following are pertinent questions: Is the current dosage excessive? Did the patient miss a meal or regular snack? Were no changes made for rigorous work or exercise? Was the injection technique correct—intramuscular vs subcutaneous (intramuscular is likely to have rapid absorption and cause possible hypoglycemia), runner or bicyclist injecting thigh vs abdomen (insulin is absorbed more rapidly from an exercising limb and should be taken in the abdominal wall in these instances)? Are reactions related to developing adrenal or pituitary insufficiency? Is the patient developing renal insufficiency? Is the diabetic taking propranolol or developing autonomic neuropathy that may mask the early adrenergic symptoms of hypoglycemia? The diabetic patient with autonomic neuropathy often loses the homeostatic/adrenergic signs and thus is at great risk for more severe hypoglycemia.

For the diabetic taking sulfonylurea agents, similar questions are appropriate: Has the patient just started on oral agents (the time when hypoglycemia with these agents is most likely to develop)? Is the patient developing renal insufficiency while taking chlorpropamide or acetohexamide—drugs that are secreted by kidneys? Is the patient taking other medication that might potentiate the hypoglycemic actions of sulfonylureas (salicylates, phenylbutazone, sulfisoxazole)? Patients who have prescriptions mistakenly filled with oral hypoglycemic agents are not rare. Always look at the pills (not just the bottle) that the patient takes with unexplained hypoglycemia. Alcohol-induced hypoglycemia develops in subjects whose livers have been depleted of glycogen. Malnourished individuals or subjects who have fasted for 48–72 hours develop hypoglycemia 6–24 hours after drinking ceases. This is typically seen in binge drinkers. These patients often present with hypothermia, coma, plasma glucose levels below 30 mg/dL, tachypnea (lactic acidosis), with or without ethanol on breath, blood ethanol levels below acute intoxication, and abnormal liver function studies. These patients do not have a hyperglycemic response when given intramuscular glucagon.

Fasting Hypoglycemia

Fasting hypoglycemias may be caused by endocrine disease (insulinomas, extrapancreatic tumors, adrenal insufficiency, pituitary insufficiency), hepatic disorders (glycogen storage disease, deficiency of gluconeogenic enzymes, acute hepatic necrosis), or, rarely, substrate deficiency in which the liver cannot produce enough glucose from lack of precursors (fasting hypoglycemia of pregnancy, ketotic hypoglycemia of childhood, uremia, and starvation). Fasting hypoglycemia is more difficult to diagnose by history than induced hypoglycemia. Because this condition is associated with significant pathology, the workup should be complete and the diagnosis definitive. By definition these patients fail to maintain plasma glucose homeostasis when food is withheld.

The most common fasting hypoglycemia is factitious. These patients have low plasma glucose and high insulin levels as do the patients with insulinoma. They surreptitiously inject insulin or ingest oral hypoglycemic agents and present for management as fasting hypoglycemia even though they really belong in the induced hypoglycemia category. Again, the differential diagnosis for any hypoglycemia is (a) medication/drug, (b) medication/drug, (c) medication/drug, and (d) other. Paramedic individuals (nurses, pharmacists, etc.) or relatives of diabetic patients are suspect for this problem. A diligent search for needle marks and of the hospital room for insulin or sulfonylureas is well worth the effort as is telephoning previous physicians and hospitals. If the patient has been injecting beef/pork insulin for several months, the serum insulin levels may appear very high (>500 U/mL) owing to antibody formation that interferes with the insulin radioimmunoassay measurement. Assaying for C peptide (the connecting peptide of proinsulin that is released in the same molar equivalents as insulin) is helpful in factitious insulin abuse where the C peptide level is low, but C peptide levels are not helpful in sulfonylurea abuse where the levels are high. Plasma/urine screening for sulfonylureas should be positive in these instances.

Patients with insulin-producing pancreatic islet adenomas (insulinomas) and tumors arising outside the pancreas classically present with fasting hypoglycemia. Insulinomas are typically seen in the middle-aged (>30 years) individual. The most important question to answer is when do the hypoglycemic symptoms occur. Headache before breakfast or the appearance of symptoms after exercise suggests fasting hypoglycemia. Weight gain often occurs because food is eaten frequently to abort or relieve the symptoms. A family history of multiple endocrine adenomatosis should be sought (about 10% of insulinomas are multiple endocrine neoplasm type 1 related).

Diagnosis of insulinoma is made when the fasting plasma glucose is low and the plasma insulin inappropriately elevated. The ratio of insulin (μU/mL) to glucose (mg/dL) is normally <0.25; a ratio of >0.3 is generally indicative of hyperinsulinism. Most patients with an insulinoma manifest hypoglycemia within 18 hours after eating. In those patients who do not manifest symptoms early and in those whose symptoms cannot be distinguished from reactive hypoglycemia, an inpatient fast of 72 hours is indicated. Ad libitum water is given and urine ketones monitored. Monitoring urine ketones is a good bedside study. It is very unlikely the patient has hyperinsulinism if the ketones are positive because insulin inhibits lipolysis. Plasma glucose and insulin are drawn every 6 hours or more often if symptoms arise. C peptide levels should be elevated with an insulinoma. Plasma glucose below 45 mg/dL and insulin above 6 μU/mL are diagnostic of hyperinsulinism.

The treatment is surgical removal of the tumor. Selective mesenteric arteriography and selective venous catheterization of the portal system looking for gradients in insulin levels help locate the tumor, but the surgeon's skill and expertise are really the most critical factors. During surgery, intraoperative sonography is particularly useful in locating nonpalpable tumors. <u>Diazoxide</u> may be tried in patients who refuse surgery or those whose hyperinsulinism is not cured by surgery. Some metastatic islet cell tumors respond to streptozotocin, but the response is unfortunately not curative.

Large mesothelial derived tumors (retroperitoneal fibrosarcomas, hemangiopericytomas), hepatomas, and adrenal carcinomas may present with fasting hypoglycemia. These tumors are large and generally easily palpable as abdominal masses. The mechanism by which the tumors cause hypoglycemia is unknown. Insulin levels are low. In some patients (40%) radioimmunoassayable insulin-like growth factor II is elevated. The tumor may overutilize glucose because of sheer bulk, but most likely some product (e.g., insulin-like growth factor II) is released that inhibits hepatic gluconeogenesis/glycogenolysis.

Antibodies to the insulin receptor typically block insulin action, leading to hyperglycemia (see immunogenic insulin resistance, page 61). However, antibodies to the insulin receptor may rarely stimulate glucose transport, leading to hypoglycemia. Other evidence of autoimmune response is also present (e.g., antinuclear antibodies, rheumatoid factor, etc.).

Postprandial Hypoglycemia

Postprandial or reactive hypoglycemia is the catch-all category characterized by hypoglycemic symptoms (adrenergic type) that develop within a few hours of eating (idiopathic reactive hypoglycemia, hereditary fructose intolerance). <u>Postprandial hypoglycemia</u> can be diagnosed when the symptoms of hypoglycemia are associated temporally with plasma glucoses below 50 mg/dL after a meal. <u>In a subset of patients who have had gastric surgery</u>, alimentary hypoglycemia appears to be due to excessive glucose loads within the duodenum, which leads to quick absorption and rapid release of insulin with resultant fall of plasma glucose to a nadir within 2.5 hours after feeding. Small frequent feedings, avoidance of foods with high simple sugar content, and judicious use of anticholinergic medication are helpful.

<u>Idiopathic or reactive hypoglycemia</u> is diagnosed using the same criteria as for postprandial hypoglycemia. The nadir occurs between 2 and 4 hours after feeding with a return to normal fasting values by the 5th and 6th hour. If there is no rebound to normal values, then a workup to exclude fasting hypoglycemia (insulinoma, adrenal or pituitary insufficiency) should be considered. The number of individuals

who have this benign syndrome of idiopathic reactive hypoglycemia is exceedingly small. These patients respond to a low carbohydrate (120 g), relatively high protein diet given as six feedings throughout the day.

Many patients make their own diagnosis of reactive hypoglycemia, attributing the symptoms of adrenergic discharge, mental and physical fatigue, and weakness that may or may not be relieved by glucose-laden food or beverage to "hypoglycemia." The lay press and media have fanned the fires by popularizing this "entity." Physicians have confused the issue themselves by not having a study that can mimic the conditions under which these patients have symptoms. The time-honored oral GTT has many problems. At least 24% of healthy inductees into the service have 2-hour plasma glucose below 60 mg/dL, and 5% have plasma glucose below 50 mg/dL without any symptoms. In a study of 650 subjects who had no symptoms before or during GTT, 10% had plasma glucose values below 47 mg/dL. The frequency of biochemical hypoglycemia is the same for patients who present for evaluation of reactive hypoglycemia as it is for the normal population. In addition most patients being evaluated for hypoglycemia with the GTT have symptoms when the corresponding plasma glucose levels are in the normal range. The 75- to 100-g load of glucose is not a physiological challenge because this is not what subjects eat at meals. These factors make interpreting the GTT results difficult. An attempt to use mixed meals (1/4–1/3 total daily calories distributed as 50% carbohydrate::20% protein::30% fat) as a challenge that might precipitate symptoms has shown that those patients who have biochemical hypoglycemia on a GTT do not have low plasma glucoses after a mixed meal yet have the same adrenergic symptoms. Thus, low plasma glucose levels cannot be confirmed to be related to 95% of patients in whom the diagnosis of reactive hypoglycemia is tentatively made. For these reasons, the author rarely orders a GTT except for screening the occasional patient for diabetes mellitus.

The hordes of patients with "nonhypoglycemic hypoglycemia" or "pseudohypoglycemia" that present to the endocrinologist's practice with the diagnosis of reactive hypoglycemia are astounding. What to say and what to recommend to these people who are looking for a handle to label their symptoms and a means of controlling these symptoms require clinical discernment. <u>For a start, ask these patients to monitor their blood glucose with a glucometer.</u> After a couple of weeks of frequent finger sticks, 95% of these patients will have convinced themselves that there is no correlation of their symptoms with blood glucoses. These patients (most often females aged 20–45) have stresses either recognized or not acknowledged. Many have chronic fatigue and somatic complaints lasting days and weeks that do not conform to typical episodic spells of true hypoglycemia. How well these patients are handling stress is reflected in the "hypoglycemic" symptoms. A tender ear and a soft tongue giving an honest assessment of the particular situation are beginning steps in managing these patients. A 120-g carbohydrate diet low in simple sugars and instructions from an innovative dietitian are helpful and should be prescribed. For the recalcitrant patient who has failed to improve despite discussion and diet, psychiatric referral may be helpful. Figure 4.1 diagrams an approach to evaluate the hypoglycemic patient.

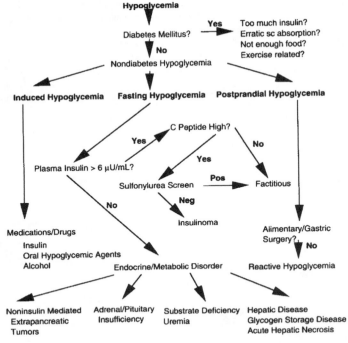

Figure 4.1. Flow diagram to evaluate patients with hypoglycemia.

Suggested Readings

Burch WM: Hypoglycemia: a handle that rarely fits. *N C Med J* 45:765, 1984.

Charles MA, Hofeldt F, Shackelford A, et al: Comparison of oral glucose tolerance tests and mixed meals in patients with apparent idiopathic postabsorptive hypoglycemia: absence of hypoglycemia after meals. *Diabetes* 30:465, 1981.

Cryer, PE: Hypoglycemia of obscure cause. *Hosp Pract* 27:119, 1992.

Hogan MJ, Service FJ, Sharbrough FW, Gerich JE: Oral glucose tolerance test compared with a mixed meal in the diagnosis of reactive hypoglycemia: a caveat on stimulation. *Mayo Clin Proc* 58:491, 1983.

Lev-Ran A, Anderson RW: The diagnosis of postprandial hypoglycemia. *Diabetes* 30:996, 1981.

Nelson RL: Hypoglycemia: fact or fiction? *Mayo Clin Proc* 60:844, 1985.

Palardy J, Havrankova J, Lepage R, et al: Blood glucose measurements during symptomatic episodes in patients with suspected postprandial hypoglycemia. *N Engl J Med* 321:1421, 1989.

Service FJ: Hypoglycemia of nondiabetic origin. In Bardin CW (ed): *Current Therapy in Endocrinology and Metabolism*, ed 4. Philadelphia, Decker, 1991, pp 359–363.

Sherwin RS, Felig P: Hypoglycemia. In Felig P, Baxter JD, Broadus AE, Frohman LA (eds): *Endocrinology and Metabolism*, ed 2. New York, McGraw-Hill, 1986, pp 1179–1202.

Chapter 5

Hyperlipidemia

Hyperlipidemia constitutes a major public concern since elevated levels of blood cholesterol are associated with premature atherosclerosis. Half of the United States population is at increased risk to develop coronary artery disease (CAD) because of hypercholesterolemia. It has not been easy to convince health professionals, patients, and the lay public of the value of hyperlipidemic therapy to prevent CAD for several reasons: (*a*) the prolonged asymptomatic period years before clinical CAD; (*b*) the customary use of a high cholesterol-saturated fat diet; and (*c*) the cost, inconvenience, and/or side effects of drugs that may produce only modest lowering of plasma lipid. However, an aggressive approach to detect and treat hyperlipidemia offers the benefit of reducing mortality and morbidity of CAD.

CHOLESTEROL AND TRIGLYCERIDES

Cholesterol and triglycerides (TG) are the major blood lipids. Each circulates bound to specific proteins (apoproteins) that function as soluble carriers and serve important roles in the metabolism of the lipids. These lipoproteins are classified as chylomicrons, low-density lipoproteins (LDL), very low-density lipoproteins (VLDL), high-density lipoproteins (HDL), and intermediate-density lipoproteins.

Blood Cholesterol

Serum or plasma total cholesterol (TC) determinations reflect the total contribution of cholesterol from LDL-cholesterol (LDL-C) (about 70% of TC), HDL-cholesterol (HDL-C) (20–25% of TC), and VLDL-cholesterol (VLDL-C) (5–10% of TC). TC comes from two sources: diet and endogenous production by the liver. One absorbs about 60% of dietary cholesterol into TG-rich chylomicrons, which are metabolized by lipoprotein lipase to chylomicron remnants, which are taken by the liver and secreted as VLDL (Fig. 5.1).

Through a cascade of metabolic processes, VLDL becomes LDL. LDL delivers cholesterol to tissues; HDL removes cholesterol from tissues. Rising levels of LDL-C favor cholesterol accumulation within tissue cells; low levels of HDL-C mean less cholesterol removal from these cells. Oxidation of LDL-C in the arterial wall leads to toxic products causing an inflammatory and proliferative response, characteristic of early atherosclerosis.

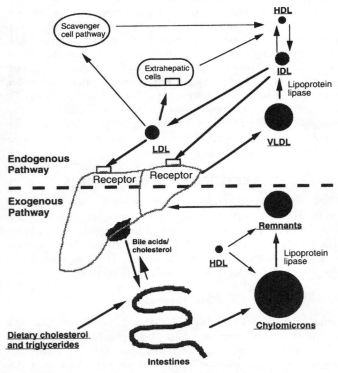

Figure 5.1. Endogenous and exogenous pathways of lipid transport. *IDL*, intermediate density lipoproteins.

Blood cholesterol levels are continuously distributed throughout the population. Levels considered normal in one geographic area may not be the same for another, with dietary intake of cholesterol and fat being the major factor. Risk for atherosclerosis increases as TC levels rise above 200 mg/dL. Blood cholesterol levels often predict CAD, but most people who have a myocardial infarction have TC that is only modestly higher than 200 mg/dL. Ratios of TC to HDL-C and LDL-C to HDL-C have been used to predict risk for CAD. Since HDL-C levels reflect "reverse transport" of cholesterol and HDL-C may act as a potent antioxidant, high levels of HDL-C (>60 mg/dL) are desirable. TC:HDL-C ratios often approach 3:1 in vegetarians. A TC:HDL-C ratio below 4:1 is considered "good." More recently, a consensus panel recommended LDL-C as the seminal marker for making treatment decisions. LDL-C can be calculated by knowing the level of TC, HDL-C, and TGs using the following formula: LDL-C = TC − (HDL-C − TG/5). LDL-C should be <130 mg/dL.

Serum Triglycerides

Serum TGs come from dietary fat (chylomicrons) and endogenous synthesis. After an overnight fast, the predominant TG circulates as <u>VLDL-TG</u> that is transported from the liver to tissues to be used as fuel or to fat for storage. Lipoprotein lipase, located in tissue capillary beds, metabolizes both chylomicrons and VLDL to chylomicron remnants and intermediate-density lipoproteins (intermediate-density lipoprotein is half TG and half cholesterol ester), respectively; the latter is atherogenic and a source for LDL-C (Fig. 5.1). Lipoprotein lipase is insulin-sensitive; any lack of insulin action leads to accumulation of TG. Again, serum TG levels, like blood cholesterol, reflect a continuous distribution; the distinction between "normal" and "abnormal" is arbitrary. Unlike blood cholesterol, mild to modest elevations of TG alone do not increase the risk of cardiovascular disease. Fasting TG levels below 250 mg/dL have no prognostic value. Values from 250 to 500 mg/dL are borderline and are often associated with secondary factors [obesity, diabetes mellitus (poorly controlled), hypothyroidism, excessive alcohol intake, renal disease (uremia, nephrotic syndrome, maintenance dialysis, and renal transplantation), liver disease, drugs (thiazide diuretics, oral contraceptives, estrogens, and some β-adrenergic blockers), glucocorticoid excess (Cushing's syndrome), and dysproteinemias]. TG levels above 500 mg/dL rep-

resent frank hypertriglyceridemia, either a primary hyperlipoproteinemia (familial) or hyperlipoproteinemia secondary to one of the
causes listed above. At these levels above 1000 mg/dL, patients are at
risk for acute pancreatitis and/or eruptive xanthoma. Furthermore,
elevated TG levels decrease HDL-C levels probably by increased hepatic clearance of HDL.

CLASSIFICATION

Most patients with increases in TC or TG do not have a single genetic
disorder but rather a sporadic, polygenic, or secondary form of hyperlipidemia. Such patients have polygenic hypercholesterolemia (20–25%
of population), combined hyperlipidemia (5–10%), and hypertriglyceridemia (10%). Although much rarer, the primary hyperlipidemias
provide models for the pathophysiology and basic understanding of
lipid metabolism. These primary hyperlipidemias include familial hypercholesterolemia, familial hypertriglyceridemia, familial combined
hyperlipidemia, familial dysbetalipoproteinemia, and chylomicronemia
syndrome. Lipoprotein phenotyping is no longer considered useful to
classify hyperlipidemia since it fails to shed any light on the pathogenesis of the disorder. For example, increased LDL levels (Type II hyperlipidemia) may be due to familial hypercholesterolemia or due to a secondary cause such as hypothyroidism or nephrotic syndrome.

Familial hypercholesterolemia, an autosomal dominant disorder, is
characterized by a deficiency or inactive cell surface LDL receptors in
the liver. The binding of LDL to its receptor forms a critical step in reg-
ulating cholesterol synthesis. Normally, this complex is internalized and
inhibits cholesterol production by decreasing hepatic hydroxymethylglu-
taryl-coenzyme A reductase activity, the rate limiting step of cholesterol
synthesis. When LDL receptors are totally deficient (homozygote), intra-
cellular cholesterol production goes unchecked, causing blood cholesterol levels of 800–1000 mg/dL. This leads to atherosclerosis by the age
of 10 years with survival rarely past 20 years. Heterozygotes (1 in 500
persons) have about half the normal number of LDL receptors and have
TC levels in the 300–450 mg/dL range. Clinically, these patients may
manifest tendon xanthoma, xanthelasma, and arcus senilis. Premature
atherosclerosis presenting as angina and/or myocardial infarction occurs between the third and fifth decade.

Familial hypertriglyceridemia, another autosomal dominant hyperlipidemia, presents with elevated VLDL-TG and rarely chylomicrons. LDL-C levels are normal. The primary defect is unknown and

is sometimes not associated with premature atherosclerosis. Family history of CAD is important in these patients.

Familial combined hyperlipidemia, another autosomal dominant trait characterized by alterations in both LDL and VLDL metabolism, may be associated with high TG or TC or both. The primary defect relates to an overproduction of VLDL and apoprotein B. This hyperlipidemia is associated with premature atherosclerosis.

Familial dysbetalipoproteinemia (Type III hyperlipoproteinemia) manifests clinically with characteristic palmar-crease xanthomas. An abnormal apoprotein E interferes with the metabolism of VLDL/intermediate-density lipoprotein and chylomicron remnants, leading to increased TG and TC. This hyperlipidemia is associated with early coronary and peripheral vascular disease.

Chylomicronemia syndrome represents severe hypertriglyceridemia associated with elevated plasma chylomicrons. The hyperchylomicronemia usually reflects a combination of a genetic and a secondary cause. Pancreatitis and eruptive xanthoma are often associated with this syndrome.

WORKUP

History

Patients at high risk for developing premature atherosclerosis include those with diabetes, hypertension, or gout and those with a family history of stroke or myocardial infarction before the age of 55. Acute or recurrent pancreatitis may be a reflection of hyperchylomicronemia. Secondary causes of hyperlipidemia are easily identified by taking an adequate history (e.g., drug-induced such as alcohol, oral contraceptives, glucocorticoids, thiazides, and β-blockers).

Physical Examination

Unfortunately, most patients with clinically significant hyperlipidemia rarely have any specific physical findings. Xanthomatosis, if present, points to certain lipid disorders. These include palmar-crease xanthoma (familial dysbetalipoproteinemia), tuberous xanthoma of Achilles tendon (familial hypercholesterolemia), eruptive xanthoma (familial or secondary hypertriglyceridemia or chylomicron syndrome). Xanthelasma, a common cutaneous manifestation of lipid deposition, is not specific for hyperlipidemia because less than half of the patients with xanthelasma have hyperlipidemia.

Laboratory Studies

An adequate assessment of the patient's lipid status requires three determinations: blood cholesterol, serum TG, and HDL cholesterol.

Blood cholesterol (TC) levels vary little throughout the day, so a random determination usually gives an accurate reflection of plasma cholesterol. Before making a diagnosis of hypercholesterolemia, at least two separate measurements should be obtained. The actual level that one calls elevated is somewhat arbitrary. Ideally, TC should be <200 mg/dL. A recent consensus panel suggests using LDL-C as the guideline lipid on which to establish treatment. LDL-C levels should be <130 mg/dL.

TG levels vary with dietary intake (e.g., chylomicron increase after a meal). If serum TGs are normal on a random sample (<250 mg/dL), then no further measurements are necessary; if elevated, then a determination after a 12-hour fast must be made. Blood obtained a few hours after an acute myocardial infarction does not accurately assess lipid status since acute illness can lower TC and raise TG. Such patients ought to have the serum lipids measured 8–12 weeks later.

HDL-C levels should also be determined. An HDL-C level below 35 mg/dL is a risk factor. It is important to know the HDL-C level because an increase in TC may be due to VLDL, LDL, or HDL.

TREATMENT

Recent studies show that atherosclerosis not only can be prevented by decreasing blood cholesterol, but atherosclerotic lesions regress when blood cholesterol is significantly lowered. These observations add renewed interest to the therapy of hyperlipidemia. Patients who have no known CAD yet have risk factors for CAD receive primary preventive treatment, whereas secondary prevention refers to patients with prior CAD and/or other atherosclerotic disease; the treatment goals are more intense in the latter group. Established positive risk factors for CAD include age (men ≥45 years; women ≥55 years or premature menopause without estrogen replacement), family history of premature coronary heart disease, hypertension, diabetes mellitus, smoking, and HDL-C below 35 mg/dL. HDL-C above 60 mg/dL is a negative risk factor for CAD. The Expert Panel of National Cholesterol Education Program uses LDL-C to make treatment decisions. Table 5.1 shows the LDL-C guidelines for initiation of dietary therapy and the goals for LDL-C on this therapy. Patients without CAD and with LDL-C of

Table 5.1
Dietary Treatment Decisions Based on LDL-C Levels

Patient Category	Initiation Level (mg/dL)	LDL Goal (mg/dL)
Without CAD		
Fewer than two risk factors	≥160	<160
Two or more risk factors	≥130	<130
With CAD	>100	≤100

≥160 mg/dL are considered high risk. Primary prevention therapy starts with diet. Patients who have CAD should initiate diet for LDL-C above 100 mg/dL with the goal to lower LDL-C below 100 mg/dL.

Dietary Therapy

Diet is the mainstay for managing hyperlipidemia regardless of type. The Step I diet recommended by the American Heart Association limits cholesterol intake to <300 mg/day, total fat calories to <30% of daily intake, and saturated fat to <10%. A Step II Diet contains <7% saturated fat and <200 mg cholesterol. For patients with fasting chylomicronemia, the total fat content should be <30 g/day. Dietary consultation with a nutritionist and/or dietitian should be obtained.

The response to diet depends on how conscientiously patients apply themselves. Faithful adherence can lower TC 10–20% and TG more. Whether this is significant depends on the starting TC level. For a patient with familial hypercholesterolemia who begins with 400 mg/dL, a 20% reduction still leaves an elevated TC (320 mg/dL). Such a patient needs pharmacotherapy. Hypolipidic agents work best in individuals who undergo diet modification because the effects are additive. Patients who are obese must lose weight and should be placed on hypocaloric diets as well. Excessive alcohol must be avoided. Patients who respond poorly to diet either may not be adhering to the diet or have a secondary disorder (e.g., poorly controlled diabetes mellitus) that needs evaluation.

Drug Therapy

Drug therapy begins with knowing the type of lipid that is primarily elevated. If the major problem is elevated LDL levels, then use drugs known to affect cholesterol metabolism. Likewise, if VLDL levels are

Table 5.2
Pharmacotherapy Based on LDL-C Levels

Patient Category	Initiation Level (mg/dL)	LDL Goal (mg/dL)
Without CAD		
Fewer than two risk factors	≥190	<160
Two or more risk factors	≥160	<130
With CAD	>130	≤100

raised, then prescribe drugs that affect TG metabolism. Drug therapy is initiated after a 3-month trial of diet fails to reach treatment goals. For hypercholesterolic patients, Table 5.2 lists the Expert Panel of National Cholesterol Education Program recommendations for initiating drug treatments and its LDL-C goal.

For low-risk men younger than 35 and premenopausal women, one can consider withholding drug therapy unless LDL-C is ≥220 mg/dL. The patient must be "sold" on the concept that lowering the lipid has positive benefits when balanced against taking lifelong medication, its side effects, and its cost. There is no ideal hypolipidemic agent. Table 5.3 lists the available agents for treating hypercholesterolemia.

Each of these drugs lowers TC by 15–25% and should be used with diet for maximal effect. Diet and bile resins offer a good starting point for most hypercholesterolemics. Minimal side effects and good efficacy make the statins (lovastatin, pravastatin, and simvastatin) a popular choice among physicians and patients; however, their long-term safety remains unknown. They inhibit hepatic hydroxymethyl-glutaryl-coenzyme A reductase activity, the rate limiting step of cholesterol synthesis. Equivalent doses are 20 mg of either lovastatin or pravastatin or 10 mg simvastatin. Doubling the dose achieves greater effects, but further dosage increases usually affect TC little. Nicotinic acid (niacin) affects the lipoprotein profile the best (lowers TC some 25% and TG up to 50% and raises HDL some 30%) and is particularly useful in those patients who have elevated TC and TG. Nicotinamide or niacinamide should not be substituted because these vitamin forms have no lipid-lowering effect. For many patients, diet plus single drug fails to control hypercholesterolemia. Combination therapy with diet, lovastatin, and another agent such as bile resin or niacin produces excellent results, often lowering TC some 50%.

Table 5.3
Drug Therapy for Hypercholesterolemia

Drug	Dose[a]	Compliance	Side Effects	Cost Per Day[b]
Statins				
Lovastatin	20–40 mg every afternoon or 40 mg bid	Good	Hepatitis, myositis	$1.60–6.30
Pravastatin	10–40 mg hs			$0.75–3.00
Simvastatin	10–40 mg hs			$1.35–5.40
Bile acid resins		Poor		
Cholestyramine	5–12 g bid		Increased VLDL levels, gastrointestinal disturbances	$1.50–2.25
Colestipol	5–15 g bid			$2.00–3.00
Nicotinic acid				
Regular	1 g tid	Fair-poor	Flushing, dyspepsia hepatic failure,	$0.50–0.75
Sustained release	750 mg bid	Good	increased uric acid and glucose	$0.50–1.00
Probucol	500 mg bid	Good	Decreased HDL levels	$2.00
Neomycin	1 g bid	Fair	Gastrointestinal disturbances, potential for otoxicity	$1.00

[a]Starting doses are lower; recheck TC in 6–8 weeks before increasing. Lovastatin, start with 20-mg tablet at evening meal; bile acid resin, start at one package or scoop bid, then 2–3 packages bid (note: take any other meds 1 hour before or 4 hours after resin dose); nicotinic acid (regular), start at 50 mg tid (1/2 of 100-mg tablet) with meals only, double at weekly intervals, later using 500-mg tablets tid (note: take one aspirin 30 min before dose to minimize side effects); nicotinic acid (sustained release), start at 250 mg with dinner for 1 week, then 250 mg bid with meals for 1 week, increasing by 250 mg/day weekly with a total daily dose of ≤250 mg; probucol, two 250-mg tablets bid with meals; neomycin, may take four 250-mg tablets hs (note: watch renal status).
[b]Cost to patient purchasing 100 tablets.

Table 5.4
Drug Therapy for Hypertriglyceridemia

Drug	Dose[a]	Compliance	Side Effects	Cost Per Day[b]
Nicotinic acid		Fair-poor	Flushing, dyspepsia, Increased uric acid	
Regular	1 g tid			$0.50–0.75
Sustained release	750 mg bid			$0.50–1.00
Gemfibrozil	600 mg bid	Good	Minimal gastrointestinal disturbances	$1.50
Clofibrate	500 mg bid	Good	Gallstones, ? overall safety	$0.80

[a]Nicotinic acid (niacin), start at 50 mg tid (half of 100-mg tablet) with meals only, double at weekly intervals, later using 500-mg tablets tid (note: take one aspirin 30 min before dose to minimize side effects); nicotinic acid (sustained release), start at 250 mg with dinner for 1 week, then 250 mg bid with meals for 1 week, increasing by 250 mg/day weekly with a total daily dose of ≤2250 mg; fish oils (10–15 g/day in divided doses) inhibit hepatic VLDL production, but must be considered investigational and may impair carbohydrate metabolism in diabetic patients.
[b]Cost to patient purchasing 100 tablets.

Certain drugs should not be used in combination such as statins (particularly lovastatin) and gemfibrozil, statins and very high-dose niacin, and statins and erythromycin. Rhabdomyolysis and renal shutdown are possible. Hepatic toxicity (transaminases) must be monitored every 6 weeks to every 4 months when administering statins and niacin, especially when these are combined. One aspirin a day is the rule for most patients. For the menopausal female, estrogen supplementation often lowers LDL-C. In addition, antioxidants are sometimes recommended for <u>adults at high risk</u> for atherosclerotic disease (β-carotene 25–30 mg/day, vitamin E 400–800 U/day, and vitamin C 500 mg/day), but their efficacy is unproven.

Patients with elevated TG (>1000 mg/dL) are at risk for developing pancreatitis and eruptive xanthomatosis. Often, a <u>secondary cause</u> can be identified and appropriate therapy reduces the TG levels. Drug therapy is ineffective in children with lipoprotein lipase deficiency, but dietary restriction of fat to <20 g/day and medium-chain length TG dietary supplements usually ameliorates the hypertriglyceridemia. Diet, weight reduction, and avoidance of alcohol often benefit adult hypertriglyceridemia. However, weight loss alone should not be relied upon as the only treatment in patients at risk for pancreatitis; patients often regain weight and need to be protected with a TG-lowering drug. Table 5.4 lists drugs that may be added to this regimen.

Once patients with hyperlipidemia are identified and treatment initiated, good follow-up is necessary after 1–4 months, depending on the intensity of diet education, medication changes, etc. One should measure TC, TG, and HDL-C on return. Appropriate changes are made if the treatment is not working. Furthermore, side effects of medication should be addressed via history and measurement of transaminases (statins, niacin, gemfibrozil) and glucose/uric acid (niacin). Effective therapy requires modification of lifestyle for most patients: diet, regular exercise, cessation of cigarette smoking, and losing weight.

Suggested Readings

Connor WE, Connor SL: Dietary treatment of hyperlipidemia: rationale and benefit. *Endocrinologist* 1:33, 1991.

Goldstein JL, Brown MS: Familial hypercholesterolemia: a genetic receptor disease. *Hosp Pract* 20:35, 1986.

Hoeg JM, Gregg RE, Brewer HB: An approach to management of hyperlipoproteinemia. *JAMA* 255:512, 1986.

Kriesberg RA: Hypercholesterolemia: dietary and pharmacotherapy. *Hosp Pract* 22:197, 1987.

Kuo PT: When and how to treat hyperlipemia. *Prim Care* 12:77, 1985.

Lavie CJ: Lipid and lipoprotein fractions and coronary artery disease. *Mayo Clin Proc* 68:618, 1993.

Patsch W, Gotto AM Jr: New perspectives on hypertriglyceridemia. *Contemp Intern Med* 5:37, 1993.

Patsch W, Patsch JR, Gotto AM Jr: The hyperlipoproteinemias. *Med Clin North Am* 73:859, 1989.

Summary of National Cholesterol Education Program Expert Panel on the Detection, Evaluation, and Treatment of High Blood Cholesterol in Adults. *JAMA* 269:3015, 1993.

Chapter 6

Pituitary Disease

Patients with pituitary-hypothalamic disorders present because of symptoms of a mass lesion (i.e., headaches, blindness, visual field defect), because of hypersecretion of a tropic hormone (prolactinoma, acromegaly, Cushing's disease), because of loss of tropic hormone(s) (hypopituitarism), or because of some combination of these.

MASS LESION

A mass lesion of the pituitary or hypothalamus should be suspected in several circumstances: (*a*) enlarged sella turcica on skull X-ray, (*b*) neurological symptoms and signs (headaches and/or loss of vision), or (*c*) endocrine disorders of the pituitary or hypothalamus.

A chance or serendipitous finding of an enlarged sella turcica on skull roentgenographs obtained for various reasons (trauma, sinusitis, headache, etc.) is not uncommon. The sella is considered enlarged if the length from the most anterior convexity to the most posterior aspect of the sella is >17 mm and if the height from the floor to a line drawn between the anterior and posterior clinoid processes is >13 mm. Other equally important roentgenographic signs are configuration of the sella, evidence of bony erosion, and presence of suprasellar calcification. If there is no obvious endocrine or visual disorder, the enlarged sella turcica may be an empty sella. Only a remnant of pituitary gland can be demonstrated by computed tomography (CT) or magnetic resonance imaging (MRI). Pituitary function studies in these patients are generally normal. Patients with primary empty sella (i.e., not a result of surgery or radiation therapy) often share some common features: female (84%), obesity (78%), hypertension (30%), benign intracranial hypertension (10%), and cerebrospinal fluid rhinorrhea (10%). Herniation of cerebrospinal fluid into the sella leads to uniform remodeling of the bone and the characteristic "ballooned" configura-

89

tion seen on lateral skull X-ray in 84% of the patients. The diagnosis of empty sella is confirmed when the CT scan or MRI identifies no mass within an enlarged sella turcica. Small coexistent tumors hypersecreting growth hormone (GH), prolactin, or adrenocorticotropic hormone (ACTH) may still be present in the sella. The patient with an empty sella who presents with cerebrospinal fluid rhinorrhea or chiasmal syndrome caused by herniation into an empty fossa is treated by conventional neurosurgical techniques as is the patient with a hyperfunctioning microadenoma (except for the prolactin-secreting adenoma). No specific therapy is needed for the empty sella.

Some mass lesions of the pituitary or hypothalamus present solely with <u>neurological symptoms</u>. The precise symptoms depend on location of the mass. Pituitary lesions are likely to cause headache as the lesion expands against the dura of the sella diaphragm. With progressive superior extension of tumor the inferior optic chiasma is compressed, leading to a visual field cut in the macula (detected by testing for color vision with a red dot—page 101), then to superior temporal field cut, then to classic bitemporal hemianopsia and eventually to blindness. Loss of visual acuity is more likely to be noticed by the patient than field cuts. Visual symptoms are less often a presenting complaint than they once were, but this is still a common mode of pituitary tumor presentation in older patients. Papilledema is rare in pituitary tumors (which usually cause optic atrophy) but is common in suprasellar tumors such as craniopharyngiomas where up to one-fourth of patients have papilledema. Craniopharyngiomas are midline, predominantly cystic tumors that develop at the upper end of the pituitary stalk. These are tumors of youth since about half of these patients are younger than 20 years. Calcification in the suprasellar region occurs in >50% of patients. Craniopharyngiomas are much more likely to compress midline hypothalamic structures, leading to neurological symptoms earlier than pituitary tumors. <u>Diabetes insipidus is common with craniopharyngiomas and rare with pituitary tumors.</u>

<u>Endocrinologic symptoms</u> are now the most common presenting complaints of patients with pituitary tumors. Hormone manifestations of pituitary tumors are caused by hypersecretion of a pituitary hormone, deficiency of pituitary hormone(s), or a combination of excess and lack of tropic hormones.

HYPERSECRETION OF A PITUITARY HORMONE

The pituitary secretes GH, gonadotropins (follicle-stimulating hormone (FSH) and luteinizing hormone (LH)), thyroid-stimulating hormone (TSH), ACTH, antidiuretic hormone (ADH), and prolactin. Many tumors may be "nonsecretory," i.e., making products that normally do not produce a distinct clinical syndrome. Examples of these tumors are the α-subunit of pituitary glycoprotein or the adenoma producing FSH.

Prolactin

Prolactin-secreting adenoma (prolactinoma), the most common pituitary tumor, causes menstrual irregularity, amenorrhea, infertility, and often galactorrhea in the female and decreased libido and impotence in the male. Excess prolactin inhibits gonadotropin secretion leading to hypogonadism. Generally there is a good correlation between tumor size and the level of serum prolactin. The diagnosis of prolactinoma is generally assured when the serum prolactin levels are >200 ng/mL. For lesser degrees of elevation one should think of prolactinoma as well as other causes of hyperprolactinemia, including drugs (estrogens, birth control pills, metoclopramide, phenothiazines, tricyclic antidepressants, opiates and opioids, cimetidine, butyrophenones, reserpine, methyl dopa, isoniazid); hypothyroidism, stress, and so forth. The MRI is the best radiographic tool for demonstrating the tumor, but small lesions (<4 mm) may not be visualized. Most prolactinomas do not stain with routine histological stains and therefore have been called chromophobe adenomas.

Treatment of prolactinoma is constantly evolving and remains controversial. Many women of childbearing age present with amenorrhea/galactorrhea as the chief complaint. These women may have microadenoma (tumor <1 cm) or no demonstrable lesion on MRI/CT. There is about a 5% chance that this tumor will progress to macroadenoma (tumor >1 cm). The major problem with these indolent microadenomas is the concomitant hypogonadism and its detrimental effect on bone. What to do for these patients depends on their desire for fertility. If there is no wish to become pregnant, then estrogen supplementation usually with oral contraceptives is prescribed. If the patient desires fertility and has a serum prolactin level of <200 ng/dL and a localized lesion on CT, there is a 90% chance that an experienced neurosurgeon using the trans-sphenoidal approach can resect the microadenoma, preserve normal pituitary function, and reduce the serum prolactin to normal. However, because of high recurrence after resection (about 25% at 5 years) and the effectiveness of medical therapy even these patients are treated with the dopamine agonist, bromocriptine, as are women who desire fertility and have no clear-cut adenoma on MRI/CT. Bromocriptine is likely to normalize prolactin levels and produce ovulation. Bromocriptine, 1.25–2.5 mg bid-tid (start 1.25 mg at bedtime to reduce nausea), is given until the pregnancy is confirmed, and then bromocriptine is discontinued. Close attention should be paid to visual fields because the pituitary lesion may occasionally enlarge during pregnancy. Patients with prolactin-secreting macroadenomas are also managed with bromocriptine unless there is evidence of visual compromise. In these cases most authorities recommend neurosurgical removal even though the chance of total extirpation of the tumor is low (<20% chance of restoring normal prolactin levels). Bromocriptine must be continued indefinitely, because once bromocriptine is stopped serum prolactin returns to existing levels before therapy. The expense for long-term administration is high ($1.25–$1.50/2.5-mg tablet); once generics are available in the United States, cost should decrease. Patient follow-up includes serum prolactin levels every 6–12 months and MRI every 1–3 years depending on clinical status.

Males with hyperprolactinemia usually have severe elevations of prolactin and often present with impotence and symptoms of a pituitary mass (macroadenoma). These patients are treated for hypogonadism if testosterone levels are low and are prescribed long-term bromocriptine. Resection of tumor may be necessary if vision is impaired.

Growth Hormone

Hypersecretion of GH leads to gigantism in children and acromegaly in adults. The changes with acromegaly are subtle, slow, and progressive for years and lead to a dramatic clinical syndrome that is not easily confused with any other syndrome. The effects of chronic hypersecretion of GH are mediated through insulin-like growth factor-I (IGF-I or somatomedin C) which causes tissue growth that is accentuated in the acral areas of the skeleton. The acral changes are most prominent in the hands where the fingers are broad and sausage-like. A handshake unmistakably suggests acromegaly in these patients. The ring size, glove size, and shoe size have enlarged over the years. The facial features are coarse with furrowed brows and prominent nasolabial creases. The cartilage of the nose hypertrophies, leading to nasal enlargement. The mandible grows, which gives an overbite, prognathism, and wide spaces between the teeth. Skin changes include skin tags, fibroma molluscum, sebaceous hypersecretion, and sebaceous cyst formation. These patients perspire more, but this decreases as activity of the disease subsides. Bone overgrowth causes hypertropic osteoarthropathy that is symptomatically difficult to treat. Carpal tunnel and other entrapment syndromes result from ligamentous hypertrophy. The liver, kidney, spleen, thyroid, and salivary glands hypertrophy. Hypertension is common and needs vigorous treatment. Overt diabetes mellitus is found in at least one-fourth of these patients. Serum T4 and testosterone levels are often low because the concentration of binding proteins for each of these hormones is lowered in acromegaly.

The diagnosis of acromegaly is confirmed by finding elevated fasting blood levels of GH (usually >10 ng/mL) that do not suppress with glucose (page 43) or are raised paradoxically in response to thyrotropin-releasing hormone (GH levels in normal subjects do not respond to thyrotropin-releasing hormone). *IGF-1* levels are also increased and correlate well with activity of the acromegaly. GH is elevated in chronic renal failure, starvation, and anorexia nervosa. Rare cases of ectopic production of GH or GH-releasing hormone have been reported in bronchial carcinoid and pancreatic islet cell tumor.

Acromegaly is treated with surgery or radiation and often with both. Therapy must be individualized for each patient and each medical center. For patients who have a well-defined lesion of <1 cm on MRI, trans-sphenoidal pituitary surgery is performed, usually with good results (GH below 2 ng/mL and normal IGF-I levels). GH-secreting tumors classically stain eosinophilic in 20% of the cases and chromophobic in the remainder of the cases. Those patients whose GH levels are >100 ng/mL have a poor response with either surgery or radiation, although GH levels may decrease dramatically and provide some clinical improvement. Conventional supervoltage irradiation delivering 4500–5000 rad to the sella through multiple ports is safe, but it takes months to years to lower GH levels. Radiation is recommended for acromegalic patients who have persistent nonsuppressible GH levels after surgery. Some patients (<20% of acromegalics) respond to bromocriptine in high doses (10–20 mg/day) and to octreotide, which must be given subcutaneously twice daily, making these quite expensive long-term therapies. Response to treatment is assessed by measuring fasting or postglucose GH and IGF-I levels.

ACTH

ACTH-producing pituitary tumors create a state of hypercortisolism that is clinically indistinguishable from other causes of glucocorticoid excess. By convention, hypercortisolism caused by bilateral adrenal hyperplasia due to a pituitary lesion is called <u>Cushing's disease</u>. Any clinical syndrome of glucocorticoid excess is called Cushing's syndrome. The <u>most common cause of Cushing's syndrome is the use of pharmacological doses of glucocorticoids</u> for various nonendocrine diseases. The differential diagnosis of hypercortisolism includes <u>Cushing's disease</u> (70–80% of the cases), <u>primary adrenal tumor</u> either adenoma or carcinoma (10–15% of the cases and, very rarely, bilateral micronodular or macronodular hyperplasia—both primary adrenal lesions), and <u>ectopic production of ACTH</u> by tumors (oat cell lung carcinomas, pancreatic islet cell carcinoma, thymoma, carcinoid tumors, medullary thyroid carcinoma, and neuroectodermal tumors). Alcoholics who have some cushingoid features and often mild degrees of hypercortisolism are diagnosed as pseudoCushing's syndrome.

Clinical signs of hypercortisolism include centripetal obesity with prominent supraclavicular fat pads, dorsal hump, and dewlap; muscle weakness and protein wasting with thin skin, facial plethora, bruising, and violaceous striae; hyperandrogenism with menstrual irregularity and hirsutism; back pain related to osteoporosis and compression fractures; hypertension particularly after the age of 40; and glucose intolerance or overt diabetes mellitus. Often, there are mental changes that include symptoms of depression, mania, psychosis, and suicide. Females are nine times more likely to have Cushing's disease than males. However, ectopic ACTH syndrome affects either sex with equal frequency.

The first question to answer is whether an obese hypertensive patient has hypercortisolism. An elevated urine cortisol establishes the diagnosis of Cushing's syndrome (pages 14–15) with about 90% accuracy. Next measure ACTH levels; normal levels are between 9 and 52 pg/mL. Values below 5 pg/mL establish the diagnosis of primary adrenal disease. An abdominal CT should be ordered, and if an adrenal mass is identified, proceed with adrenalectomy. If the ACTH level is elevated, there is about a 90% chance of pituitary-dependent adrenal hyperplasia and a 10% probability of ectopic ACTH production (nonpituitary source). Most patients with ectopic ACTH production present not with classical stigmata of Cushing's (obesity, striae, etc.) but with weakness, weight loss, and hypokalemic alkalosis; often the malignancy is known, frequently small cell lung carcinoma. That leaves Cushing's disease as the most likely cause of hypercortisolism.

ACTH-producing pituitary tumors are small, often <5 mm; thus they are not detected by skull X-ray and are detected only half of the time with high resolution CT or MRI scan. Symptoms of Cushing's syndrome lead to evaluation early in the disease, accounting for the infrequent radiographic findings. However, confirming this diagnosis is not always easy; in fact, I called Cushing's syndrome a "humbling" disease. It occasionally humbles the physician making the diagnosis and pinpointing the source. The problem is the rare patient who may demonstrate excessive amounts of cortisol intermittently or periodically such that the overnight dexamethasone study and urine free cortisol are normal. Then a few patients with "occult" ectopic ACTH production, such as those with an indolent bronchial carcinoid, may mimic pituitary-dependent adrenal hyperplasia. Remember the MRI of the pituitary in Cushing's disease is often normal or has minor changes seen in 10–15% of the normal population, so the MRI often is nondiagnostic or leads one down the wrong road (assuming that the pituitary lesion is the source of ACTH when it is not).

Traditionally, dexamethasone suppression studies are used to separate etiologies of the hypercortisolism (page 15). Patients with Cushing's disease suppress their adrenal steroid output as a result of ACTH suppression by high dose dexamethasone; patients with adrenal tumors and ectopic ACTH syndrome do not. Biochemical studies including high-dose dexamethasone and metyrapone loading may suggest a pituitary origin (e.g., >50% suppression with dexamethasone), but on occasion a patient has ectopic ACTH production as the source. Studies that aid localization of the ACTH include corticotrope-releasing hormone (CRH) infusion and sampling of the venous effluent from the pituitary for ACTH via bilateral petrosal vein or cavernous sinus catheterization. Administrating CRH improves the accuracy of the diagnosis to 90%, but if the pretest probability is 90% Cushing's disease in ACTH-dependent hypercortisolism, there is not much to gain from doing such a study. Petrosal sinus catheterization combined with CRH infusion that produces a 2- to 3-fold increase in ACTH localizes the process to the pituitary. This "gold standard study" has some problems. It is invasive and costly ($2500); CRH is not generally available in the United States; and only a few centers have radiologists experienced enough to routinely recommend catheterization of pituitary venous outflow for determination of ACTH gradients. By using stricter criteria for high dose dexamethasone study (suppression to 90% of baseline urine free cortisol and 65% of baseline 17-OHCS), one can feel confident that the pituitary is the source of ACTH. If the classical Liddle suppression test is clearly suggestive of a primary pituitary problem and if a chest MRI shows no abnormality, I recommend pituitary surgery in such patients. When the data are less clear or previous surgery has failed to cure the hypercortisolism, then I proceed with catheterization studies. Remember the patient who most likely has an ectopic source of ACTH is a male often with high levels of ACTH (>400 pg/mL).

In the past the only effective treatment of Cushing's disease was to remove the hypertrophied adrenal glands, leaving the patient permanently dependent on replacement glucocorticoid and mineralocorticoid. Significant hyperpigmentation and sella enlargement caused by a large ACTH-producing tumor (Nelson's syndrome) follows adrenalectomy in about 8% of the cases. Trans-sphenoidal pituitary microsurgery, which cures 75–95% of patients while preserving pituitary function, is the therapy of choice. Ninety-five percent of Cushing's disease patients have an adenoma; the remainder have basophil/corticotrope hyperplasia. Here as in other endocrine surgery, an experienced surgeon is critical for optimum results. Sometimes total anterior hypophysectomy is performed when the microadenoma cannot be found. Patients who are cured of the Cushing's are hypoadrenal in the immediate postoperative period. By 48–72 hours, plasma cortisols are low, and symptoms of hypocortisolism such as nausea and vomiting are evident. These patients need glucocorticoid supplementation for months to 1–2 years until the hypothalamic-pituitary-adrenal axis has recovered from the suppressive effects of prolonged exposure to excessive glucocorticoids. If the patient is not hypoadrenal postoperatively, the surgery failed. Recurrence of Cushing's disease after successful pituitary surgery ranges from 5 to 20%, so "cured" patients need good follow-up. Bilateral adrenalectomy still has a role for those patients not cured with pituitary surgery, some patients with recurrent Cushing's disease, or those patients in whom the pituitary technically cannot be approached trans-sphenoidally (e.g., venous plexus in front of the pituitary gland). For patients whose source of ectopic ACTH cannot be found, control of hypercortisolism may be achieved medically by taking ketoconazole ± metyrapone. In children with Cushing's disease the treatment of choice has been pituitary irradiation, but trans-sphenoidal pituitary surgery appears equally effective.

DEFICIENCY OF TROPIC HORMONES

Loss of tropic hormones leading to hypopituitarism is common in pituitary disorders. There are numerous and diverse causes, including processes that may affect the pituitary directly by leading to primary hypopituitarism (e.g., pituitary adenoma or hemorrhage) or indirectly by disturbing hypothalamus or stalk functions, leading to secondary hypopituitarism (e.g., sarcoid). Table 6.1 lists most causes of hypopituitarism.

Clinical signs and symptoms of hypopituitarism relate to the underlying cause and to the specific tropic hormone(s) that are missing. Onset is usually insidious, but occasionally the presentation is dramatic as with acute diabetes insipidus or pituitary apoplexy. Mass le-

Table 6.1
Causes of Hypopituitarism

Primary	Secondary
Pituitary tumors	**Destruction of stalk**
Intrasellar and parasellar	Trauma
	Compression by mass
Infarction or ischemic necrosis	Surgical trans-section
Postpartum (Sheehans' syndrome)	
Shock	**Hypothalamic disease**
Sickle cell anemia	Inflammation (sarcoidosis,
Cavernous sinus thrombosis	eosinophilic granuloma)
Carotid artery aneurysm or thrombosis	Trauma
Pituitary apoplexy	Toxic (vincristine)
Diabetes mellitus	Hormone-induced (high
	glucocorticoids)
Inflammatory disease	Tumors
Meningitis (tuberculosis, fungal,	Functional
malarial)	Starvation
Pituitary abscess	Anorexia nervosa
	Psychosocial dwarfism
Infiltrative disorders	
Hemochromatosis	
Idiopathic	
Selective hormone deficiency	
Isolated GH deficiency	
Isolated ACTH deficiency	
Isolated thyroid-stimulating hormone	
Hypogonadotropic hypogonadism	
Multiple hormone deficiency	
Iatrogenic	
Irradiation to sella or nasopharynx	
Surgical destruction	

sions compress and distort normal pituicytes, leading to loss of tropic hormones. The tropic hormone usually lost first is <u>GH</u>, followed by the <u>gonadotropins</u>, and finally by <u>TSH</u> and <u>ACTH</u>. ADH deficiency is rare with pituitary disease but is common with stalk and hypothalamic lesions.

GH deficiency is not clinically detectable in the adult. In children GH deficiency leads to growth failure and short stature and, rarely, to hypoglycemia. Likewise gonadotropin deficiency causes no symptoms in the postmenopausal or posthysterectomy female. Absence of FSH and LH produces hypogonadism with amenorrhea and infertility in adult females and impotence in adult males. Hypothyroidism secondary to TSH deficiency and hypoadrenalism secondary to ACTH deficiency are late complications of pituitary tumor. Patients with these deficiencies often present with a mass lesion and neurological symptoms related to loss of vision. Isolated tropic hormone deficiency is usually diagnosed in youth because of failure to grow or failure to enter puberty.

EVALUATION OF PITUITARY FUNCTION

Several studies are necessary to assess pituitary function: baseline or static studies, dynamic or provocative testing, visual assessment, and radiographic studies.

Baseline Studies

Serum taken for one determination detects absolute deficiencies in some circumstances. For example, serum testosterone and LH are ordered in the evaluation of the impotent male. If both testosterone and LH are low, then these static studies establish the diagnosis of secondary hypogonadism. To completely evaluate the etiology of the hypogonadism several questions must be addressed: (a) Are there other tropic hormone deficiencies? (b) Is the serum prolactin elevated (prolactin suppresses gonadotropin)? (c) Is there a mass lesion (abnormal sella turcica, compromised visual fields, enhanced lesion on MRI/CT scan)? If not, consider hemochromatosis or other infiltrative disease.

Table 6.2 lists static studies that may be ordered to assess deficiencies of pituitary hormones. ACTH normally has peaks and valleys throughout the day, so a low ACTH level alone is not helpful. ACTH can be assessed indirectly by a 24-hour urine cortisol; TSH can be assessed by serum T4/T3U or free T4 and ADH by an early morning urine specific gravity. If any value is low in a patient with obvious pi-

Table 6.2
Static Studies to Assess Pituitary Function

Tropic Hormone	Study to Order	Value If Hypopituitary
GH	Plasma GH	Low or normal (high in anorexia nervosa)
LH	If amenorrhea, serum LH	Low LH
	If male, serum testosterone and LH	Low testosterone–low LH
FSH	Serum FSH in women	Low FSH
	Semen analysis and FSH for men	Low sperm count and semen volume
TSH	T4(RIA)/T3U or free T4; TSH	Low T4 and T3U; low TSH
ACTH	24-hour urine free cortisol	Low
Prolactin	Serum prolactin	High (if prolactinoma)
ADH	Early morning urine specific gravity	Specific gravity <1.005

LH, luteinizing hormone; FSH, follicle-stimulating hormone; TSH, thyroid-stimulating hormone; T4, thyroxine.

tuitary disease, one can assume a deficiency for the appropriate tropic hormone. Serum prolactin should be determined.

Dynamic Testing

Serum or urine hormone concentration measured under stimulatory conditions assesses whether there is reserve for the respective hormone and ascertains whether the patient can tolerate surgical procedures or other stress situations. Dynamic studies such as the insulin-induced hypoglycemia or metyrapone loading are not necessary in the patient with an obvious mass lesion. These studies are conducted primarily when there are questions about whether there is any pituitary disease or dysfunction. In these patients, the insulin-induced hypoglycemia test is an ideal stimulatory study since both GH and cortisol can be measured (page 9). In practice, dynamic studies for pituitary hypofunction are less frequently performed now. In the past, physicians were armed with only a skull X-ray, pneumoencephalogram, and visual testing to detect pituitary disease; subtle pituitary disease might be detected with dynamic testing. Today, radiography with MRI and/or CT detects structural changes and allows follow-up. Of the dynamic studies, I use the short cosyntropin study to assess ACTH-adrenal reserve (page 11) and, less often, GnRH testing.

Visual Assessment

Visual acuity and visual fields should be assessed at the bedside. Testing visual acuity is important (a hand-held chart works fine) and is a parameter that should not be neglected. The most reliable method for testing visual fields is based on the patient's ability to count fingers shown by the examiner (Fig. 6.1). The examiner asks the patient to look directly into the examiner's own pupil, which allows comparison of the patient's visual field with that of the observer. With one eye occluded, either <u>one</u>, <u>two</u>, or <u>five fingers</u> are presented in each of four quadrants of the visual field in different positions, and the patient is asked to give the correct number of fingers. Showing three and four fingers is confusing and should be avoided. Most fibers in the optic chiasm derive from the central portion of the visual field, and these axons subserve color vision. For this reason central visual fields are the first to be affected by expanding sellar tumors and can be tested using bright red objects (Fig. 6.2).

The patient fixates on the examiner's eye and is asked to compare the brightness of color of two objects, one held in the temporal field and the other held in the nasal field. Both objects are held together close to the line of fixation (central vision). In the case of a chiasmal lesion, the patient will be unable to distinguish the red color in the

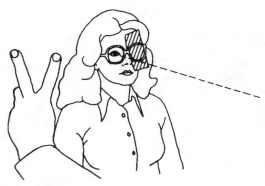

Figure 6.1. Assessing vision fields by confrontation. With one eye occluded, patient fixates gaze on examiner's pupil. Examiner asks patient to enumerate one, two, or five fingers presented in each quadrant. This examination is repeated with other eye. (From Neelon FA, Syndor CF. The assessment of pituitary function. *Disease-a-Month* 24:20, 1978.)

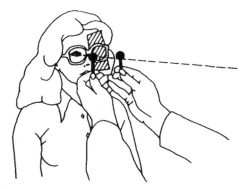

Figure 6.2.   Assessing central vision fields by color confrontation. One eye is occluded, and patient fixates gaze on examiner's pupil. Two bright objects (such as red paper or bottle caps) are presented on both sides of fixation. Patient is asked to compare presence and brightness of color. (From Neelon FA, Syndor CF. The assessment of pituitary function. *Disease-a-Month* 24:20, 1978.)

temporal field or will note that the test object is much redder in the nasal than in the temporal field.

Visual field examination performed by perimetry (e.g., Goldmann apparatus) is important as a baseline study and is the procedure of choice for detecting minor visual field abnormalities and for following changes in visual fields.

Radiographic Studies

CT and MRI scans have replaced the pneumoencephalogram in evaluation of mass lesions. Both studies give similar resolution of mass or tumor size. The CT identifies bony invasion (bone shows well on CT) such as pituitary tumor extending anteriorly into the sphenoid sinus or meningioma attached to bone. The MRI shows vascular tissue and gives great detail of white and gray matter. Patients allergic to radiographic contrast dyes are ideal candidates for MRI because these agents are not used in MRI. The MRI helps define lateral extension of pituitary tumor into the cavernous sinuses and superior extension against the optic nerve (which is well seen on MRI). In addition, MRI shows the anatomy of the carotid vessels (e.g., "kissing" carotid arteries), so angiography or digital subtraction angiography can be avoided. Of the two studies (CT vs MRI), MRI with gadolium is better.

MANAGING HYPOPITUITARY PATIENT DURING SURGICAL PROCEDURES
General Surgery

Hypopituitary patients require exogenous glucocorticoids during and after surgery. There are several regimens to provide glucocorticoids for the stress of surgery and anesthesia. The most frequently used method is to give hydrocortisone succinate (Solu-Cortef) 100 mg as an <u>intravenous drip</u> every 6–8 hours during surgery and taper the dose over a few days after the operation until oral medications are well tolerated. Another regimen that does not depend on continuous infusions is intramuscular cortisone acetate by the following schedule: 100 mg into *each* buttock 2 days before surgery and on the day before surgery (200 mg/day) and 100 mg im on call to the operating room. Cortisone acetate 100 mg im is given daily until oral medications are tolerated. If there is hypothermia (e.g., cardiac bypass surgery) or hypotension, then intravenous administration is the preferable route.

When the patient is stable (e.g., no fever, infection, etc.) and can take oral medications, then oral hydrocortisone 20 mg tid or cortisone acetate 25 mg bid is given until discharge from the hospital. Maintenance glucocorticoid therapy consists of hydrocortisone 20–30 mg/day in divided doses bid to tid or cortisone acetate 25–37.5 mg/day bid (before breakfast and evening meal).

If the preoperative evaluation demonstrates the patient to be hypothyroid, surgery need not be postponed. Doses of analgesic medications are reduced to accommodate the decreased metabolism, and replacement L-thyroxine is begun, starting at a dose of 25 μg/day for 2–3 weeks, increased to 50–100 μg/day for 2–3 weeks, and then maintained at 75–150 μg/day (1.7 μg/kg body weight/day).

Pituitary Surgery

Patients scheduled for pituitary surgery should have these baseline endocrine studies performed: prolactin, FSH and LH, free T4 or T4/T3U, morning urine specific gravity, serum testosterone (if male), and GH and IGF-I (if acromegaly suspected). Patients with microadenoma and no clinical evidence for hypopituitarism need no special endocrine supplementation. Patients with large pituitary tumors should be given intravenous hydrocortisone intraoperatively

(Solu-Cortef 100 mg every 6 hours), which should be continued for 48 hours after the operation. If the surgeon noted normal pituitary tissue that was not perturbed by surgery, then discontinue hydrocortisone altogether at 48 hours. Twenty-fours after the last dose of hydrocortisone, obtain blood for a plasma cortisol level. If the plasma cortisol is >9 μg/dL, then the patient may be safely discharged on no glucocorticoid supplementation. If the plasma cortisol is <3 μg/dL, these patients are invariably hypoadrenal and need lifelong hydrocortisone treatment. Cortisol values between 3 and 9 μg/dL are indeterminate in regard to permanent hypoadrenalism, so these patients are discharged on maintenance hydrocortisone/cortisone acetate. In follow-up 4–6 weeks later, these patients should omit their morning dose of steroids on the day of the clinic visit. A short cosyntropin study is performed (page 11). If plasma cortisol rises to >18 μg/dL, then the oral glucocorticoids can be discontinued altogether. Less than a normal response means staying on maintenance steroids. This is an excellent time to assess thyroid and gonadal status and check levels of the hypersecretory product (e.g., prolactin, GH) if that was the reason for the surgery.

A significant increase in urine output immediately after pituitary surgery usually indicates diabetes insipidus, but diabetes mellitus must be excluded. Replacement with intravenous fluid in amounts equivalent to urine output is justified for several hours. Then reduce the intravenous rate for 1–2 hours and check the serum and urine osmolality. A plasma osmolality above 287 mOsm/kg ensures volume contraction and excludes volume overload as the cause of the diuresis. Aqueous vasopressin 5 U sc is given. If the patient has diabetes insipidus, both urine volume and serum osmolality should decrease over the next hour in response to vasopressin. The diabetes insipidus may be transient or permanent. Give subcutaneous aqueous pitressin or desmopressin every 6–12 hours as required if excessive urine output (arbitrarily >200 mL/hour) is accompanied by increased thirst. One should be aware of the triphasic response of diuresis-antidiuresis-diuresis after pituitary or hypothalamic injury. One to two days after the operation there is a diuresis that lasts 3–5 days (probably caused by neurohypophyseal trauma), then amelioration for 4–5 days (caused by release of stored ADH granules), followed by full-blown diuresis (the sequela of permanent injury). After the diagnosis of diabetes insipidus is firmly established, one prescribes desmopressin. If the thirst mechanism is intact, as it usually is, then taking vasopressin is a matter of convenience to avoid having to drink excessively and urinate frequently. Desmopressin is taken 0.05–0.15 mL once to twice per day and administered intranasally by blowing the solution out of a cannula directed into the nares or using a nasal spray that squirts 0.1 mL for each puff. Cost of desmopressin is a factor ($60.00 for 2.5 mL with average expense $1750–2500/year). Lysine vasopressin (Diapid) nasal spray is effective but must be used at frequent intervals (every 3–6 hours). Pitressin tannate-in-oil is no longer available.

Postoperative radiation of the sella is usually prescribed for patients with large tumors because it is rare to completely remove all tumor during surgery. These patients are usually continued on maintenance glucocorticoids during and after radiation. To determine whether a patient who was placed on postoperative prophylactic steroids needs lifelong treatment, ask the patients to hold their afternoon hydrocortisone the evening before and the morning hydrocortisone on the day of clinic visit. Measure baseline plasma cortisol and perform the short cosyntropin study. If the plasma cortisol rises to >18 μg/dL, then glucocorticoids are discontinued. If the baseline value is <5 μg/dL and the stimulated cortisol is <18 μg/dL, there is not much chance for successful withdrawal, and the patient should continue maintenance replacement. <u>Patients should double or triple their maintenance glucocorticoid dose during episodes of stress (fever, flu, diarrhea, minor surgery, etc.).</u> Some form of identification (Medic-Alert) noting the diagnosis of hypopituitarism and steroid dependence should be worn.

Hypogonadal men need replacement androgen to preserve libido and potency as well as to maintain muscle mass and stamina. Testosterone given as testosterone cypionate 200 mg im (Depo-Testosterone) or testosterone enanthate 200 mg im (Delatestryl) every 2–4 weeks is the best choice. Intramuscular testosterone has many advantages: it is effective and inexpensive; serum levels are maintained for at least 2 weeks after injection; and one avoids the complication of cholestatic hepatitis that is occasionally seen with oral androgens.

SYNDROME OF INAPPROPRIATE ADH SECRETION

Under normal circumstances, the hypothalamus senses serum osmolality and regulates serum tonicity within well-defined limits by the interaction of the thirst center and the release or inhibition of release of ADH. When the serum osmolality rises, ADH is released. Renal tubules respond by increasing the resorption of water, and the thirst center responds by giving the sensation of thirst. Both actions decrease serum osmolality. Furthermore, decreased vascular volume (e.g., de-hydration, hypovolemia, or hypotension) enhances ADH secretion. Volume status is a much stronger physiologic stimulus for ADH release and takes precedent over osmolality (even when serum osmolality is low; a state when ADH secretion is normally inhibited). The syndrome of inappropriate ADH (SIADH) exists whenever there is ADH secre-tion in the presence of low plasma osmolality and in the absence of states that cause ADH secretion such as hypovolemia. Continual ADH secretion leads to decreased free water clearance and dilutional hy-ponatremia. Diagnosis of SIADH should be suspected when there is a combination of hyponatremia (serum sodium usually <130 mEq/L) and an inappropriately concentrated urine (often >300 mOsm/kg). Urine sodium is usually >20 mEq/L in SIADH, which is inappropri-ate for patients who are taking normal amounts of salt. This is in con-trast to patients with hyponatremia with decreased effective blood vol-ume (e.g., heart failure, ascites) where renal tubular resorption of sodium is increased and the urine sodium is <20 mEq/L. There are multiple causes of SIADH: (*a*) ectopic production of ADH (SIADH was first described in patients with bronchogenic carcinoma, which re-mains the most common cause of this syndrome); (*b*) central nervous system disorders (head injuries, vascular lesions, infections, Guillain-Barré syndrome, and acute intermittent porphyria); (*c*) drugs (vin-cristine, chlorpropamide, carbamazepine); and (*d*) endocrine disease (Addison's disease, hypothyroidism). The clinical features are weight gain and symptoms of hyponatremia (weakness, lethargy, and mental confusion). Seizures are treated with intravenous hypertonic saline (5%) in amounts to increase the serum sodium to 120 mEq/L. All SIADH patients are volume replete and need restriction of fluids to <1000 mL/day. Sodium loading is not helpful since these patients re-spond by excreting it into the urine without correcting the hypona-tremia. If fluid restriction does not work or the underlying disorder cannot be treated effectively (e.g., oat cell carcinoma of the lung), then administration of demeclocycline 300 mg tid to qid to inhibit action of ADH on the renal tubule may prove effective.

Suggested Readings

Burch W: A survey of results with transsphenoidal surgery in Cushing's dis-ease. *N Engl J Med* 308:103, 1983.

Flack MR, Oldfield EH, Cutler GB Jr, et al: Urine free cortisol in high-dose dexamethasone suppression test for differential diagnosis of Cushing syn-drome. *Ann Intern Med* 116:211, 1992.

Frohman LA: Diseases of anterior pituitary. In Felig P, Baxter JD, Broadus AE, Frohman LA (eds): *Endocrinology and Metabolism,* ed 2. New York, McGraw-Hill, 1986, pp 247–337.

Gold EM: The Cushing's syndromes: changing views of diagnosis and treatment. *Ann Intern Med* 90:829, 1979.

Jordan RM, Kendall JW, Kerber CW: The primary empty sella. *Am J Med* 62:569, 1977.

Meikle AW: A diagnostic approach to Cushing's syndrome. *Endocrinologist* 3:311, 1993.

Molitch ME, Elton RL, Blackwell RE, et el: Bromocriptine as primary therapy for prolactin-secreting macroadenomas: results of a prospective multicenter study. *J Clin Endocrinol Metab* 60:698, 1985.

Schlechte J, Sherman B, Halmi N, et al: Prolactin-secreting pituitary tumors in amenorrheic women: a comprehensive study. *Endocr Rev* 1:295, 1980.

Streeten DHP, Moses AM: The syndrome of inappropriate vasopressin secretion. *Endocrinologist* 3:353, 1993.

Tahir AH, Sheeler LR: Recurrent Cushing's disease after transsphenoidal surgery. *Arch Intern Med* 152:977, 1992.

Thapar K, Kovacs K, Laws ER Jr, Muller PJ: Pituitary adenomas: current concepts in classification, histopathology, and molecular biology. *Endocrinologist* 3:39, 1993.

Watts NB, Tindall GT: Rapid assessment of corticotropin reserve after pituitary surgery. *JAMA* 259:708, 1988.

Vance ML: When bromocriptine fails. *Endocrinologist* 1:119, 1991.

Chapter 7

Amenorrhea

Menstrual dysfunction is frequent in many disorders. The absence of menses is normal before puberty, during pregnancy, and after ovarian function ceases (menopause). Normal menstruation depends on normal anatomy and physiology: (*a*) patent outlet (normal vagina and cervix); (*b*) uterus that responds to estrogen and progesterone stimulation; (*c*) ovaries that respond to gonadotropins with estrogen and progesterone production; and (*d*) the pituitary and hypothalamus, which sense the hormone milieu and respond with release of gonadotropins. <u>Amenorrhea, defined as absence of menstruation in any female older than 16 years (primary amenorrhea) or absence of menses for >6 months in a woman of childbearing age with a history of menstruation (secondary amenorrhea), requires evaluation.</u> The diagnostic workup begins with the history and physical examination in an attempt to segregate which organ abnormality is causing the amenorrhea: outlet tract, uterus, ovary, or central nervous system (pituitary and hypothalamus). Localizing the cause(s) of amenorrhea often presents a challenge.

<u>Age</u>, <u>history</u>, and <u>physical examination</u> give helpful clues regarding etiology. Pubertal age females with amenorrhea are more likely to have outlet abnormalities and ovarian dysgenesis, whereas older women with amenorrhea who have had prior menses are more likely to have pituitary-hypothalamic disorders. A history of weight loss, amenorrhea, bulimia, and bradycardia in a otherwise healthy teenager suggests <u>anorexia nervosa</u>. <u>Postpartum amenorrhea</u> and the inability to nurse may be secondary to pituitary hemorrhage (Sheehan's syndrome). Amenorrhea caused by destruction of the endometrium (Asherman's syndrome) and scarification as a result of overzealous postpartum curettage should also be considered. <u>Physical examination</u> identifies most causes of primary amenorrhea (listed in order of decreasing frequency): (*a*) <u>Turner's syndrome</u> (gonadal dys-

genesis) with sexual infantilism (absent breast development) and its somatic manifestations (short stature, webbed neck, widely spaced nipples, etc.); (*b*) <u>congenital absence of vagina</u> with normal growth and sexual development (breast, pubic and axillary hair, feminine figure); (*c*) <u>testicular feminization</u> with blind vaginal pouch, scant pubic hair, inguinal hernia, and often palpable inguinal masses; and (*d*) <u>imperforate hymen</u>. Galactorrhea with amenorrhea indicates a pituitary abnormality (possible prolactinoma). Amenorrhea may relate to underlying chronic disease (hepatic and renal failure) or to other endocrine disorders such as thyroid disease (hyperthyroidism and hypothyroidism), adrenal disease (hypocortisolism and hypercortisolism), and hirsutism.

WORKUP

When the diagnosis is not evident from the history and physical examination and pregnancy is excluded (serum β-HCG or urine for chorionic gonadotropin is negative), the following studies are performed: (*a*) **serum prolactin** to assess whether hyperprolactinemia is the cause of the secondary amenorrhea; (*b*) **serum gonadotropins (follicle-stimulating hormone (FSH) and luteinizing hormone (LH))** to determine if there is primary ovarian failure; and (*c*) **progestin administration** to assess the level of endogenous estrogen and the competence of outlet tract. Medroxyprogesterone acetate (Provera), 10 mg po every day for 5 days, is given. Vaginal bleeding should occur within 1 week after Provera is discontinued. Withdrawal bleeding indicates normal endogenous estrogen levels because proliferative endometrium (which is under estrogenic stimulation) must be present if Provera is to have an effect (progesterone converts proliferative into a secretive endometrium). Withdrawal bleeding will not occur in <u>outlet obstruction</u> (congenital absent vagina), <u>uterine agenesis</u> (testicular feminization, XY gonadal dysgenesis), <u>endometrial scarring</u> (Asherman's syndrome), or in the <u>"unprimed" uterus</u> as in low estrogen states (gonadal failure, hypopituitarism). Patients who have withdrawal bleeding and normal serum prolactin levels have <u>anovulation</u> as the etiology of their amenorrhea (polycystic ovarian disease, extraglandular estrogen formation, psychogenic causes). Patients with elevated prolactin levels need brain CT and/or MRI to evaluate for mass lesions of the pituitary (page 89). Figure 7.1 shows a flow diagram to evaluate amenorrhea.

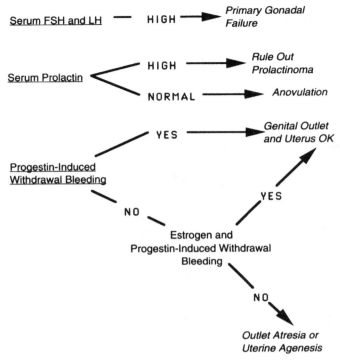

Figure 7.1.   Flow diagram to evaluate amenorrhea.

An additional study to perform in women who do not have withdrawal bleeding after medroxyprogesterone administration is to prime the endometrium with conjugated estrogen (Premarin 1.25 mg bid for 21 days) followed by progesterone (Provera 10 mg every day for 5 days). Withdrawal bleeding does not occur in <u>outlet obstruction or end-organ abnormality</u> (uterine agenesis or Asherman's syndrome). Females with <u>testicular feminization</u> fail to have withdrawal bleeding because no uterus is present. These women represent a classic example of hormone resistance, in this case, androgen-resistance. Testicular feminization is inherited as an X-linked recessive trait. The genotype is XY although the phenotype is unmistakably female. These young women present with primary amenorrhea, normal growth and development, and have well-developed secondary sex features (breasts and feminine figure). The skin and its appendages are not stimulated by normal or high normal levels of serum testosterone, leading to little to no axillary or pubic hair. Testes are present in the inguinal canal or are within the abdomen. These gonads are removed because their incidence of neoplasia approaches 50% in women older than 30.

Withdrawal bleeding after therapy with estrogen-progesterone confirms the presence of a uterus that responds to hormone stimulation and localizes the abnormality to either the ovary or the pituitary-hypothalamus. The gonadotropins, FSH and LH, are elevated in gonadal failure. FSH values of >40 mIU/mL are diagnostic of primary gonadal failure. LH levels are elevated before ovulation and are not as specific for gonadal failure as raised FSH levels. Patients with typical Turner's syndrome have short stature (rarely >58 inches), stocky build, webbed neck, widely spaced nipples ("shield chest"), and cubitus valgus. These patients have the 45,XO genotype, but mosaicism is common (XO/XX). Any hypergonadotropic patient <35 years old with primary amenorrhea needs karyotyping to exclude the presence of Y chromosome because the incidence of malignant tumors developing within dysgenetic gonads is about 25%; gonadectomy is necessary for these patients.

Premature menopause occurs much earlier than average age of menopause (range 45–55 years), is associated with elevated FSH and LH levels, and may be due to surgical oophorectomy, autoimmune oophoritis (e.g., associated with polyglandular failure), radiation to the pelvis, or chemotherapy. If the serum LH is <5 mIU/mL, then hypopituitarism is likely.

MANAGEMENT

Treatment of the amenorrhea is directed to the specific cause. Surgical correction of anatomical abnormalities such as imperforate hymen, congenital agenesis of vagina, and endometrial scarring are generally successful. Hypogonadism caused by primary ovarian failure is treated with estrogen therapy. Replacement therapy should be tailored to fit individual patient needs. Commonly used estrogens are listed in Table 7.1.

Women who have gonadectomy for Y chromosome genotype (gonadal dysgenesis or testicular feminization) or those who have surgical oophorectomy or premature menopause need estrogen supplementation. For the premenopausal women who have a uterus, se-

Table 7.1
Equivalent Doses of Estrogens Used for Replacement

Estrogen	Brand	Dose	Cost Per Month
Conjugated equine estrogens	Premarin	0.625 mg	$9
Piperazine estrone sulfate	Ogen	0.625–1.25 mg	$11
Micronized estradiol-17β	Estrace	1.0 mg	$11
Transdermal estradiol-17β	Estraderm	0.05 mg	$17–19

quential estrogen-progesterone is prescribed either as oral contraceptives or conjugated equine estrogens (Premarin 1.25–2.5 mg every day) for 25 days followed by medroxyprogesterone acetate (Provera) 5–10 mg on days 16–25. Beginning medication on the first day of every month establishes an easily remembered routine. Menstruation usually begins on the 27th day of each month. The estrogen dose needs to be increased (up to 10 mg Premarin/day) in pubertal females to achieve secondary sex characteristics (breast development and more feminine appearance). Estrogen dose should be decreased in patients who complain of fluid retention.

For the menopausal and postmenopausal female who have not had a hysterectomy, several options are possible: sequential estrogen-progestin as above, concomitant daily estrogen-progestin such as Premarin 0.625 mg/Provera 2.5 mg (which after a few months leads to atrophic endometrium and thus absent menses—a plus for most women), or transdermal estrogen patch with Provera 5–10 mg on days 16–25 or continuous daily Provera 2.5 mg. Transdermal estrogen patch must be changed every 3 days, has a theoretical advantage of bypassing the liver and thus avoiding the effects on synthesis of several hepatic proteins seen with oral estrogens, and is about twice as expensive as the most commonly prescribed oral estrogen (Premarin). For hysterectomized women, progestin treatment is not necessary, only estrogen.

Secondary hypogonadism is managed as far as the underlying disorder can be corrected (e.g., surgery for a pituitary tumor or bromocriptine for prolactinoma). Chronic anovulation related to polycystic ovarian disease is usually treated with oral contraceptives in an attempt to suppress androgen production (page 125). Other endocrine diseases associated with anovulation (e.g., Cushing's syndrome, Addison's disease, thyrotoxicosis, hypothyroidism) should be treated first. Exercise-induced amenorrhea seen in athletes leads to decreased bone mineral content, often at a critical time when final bone mass is developing. This osteopenia is usually not reversible, so estrogen replacement should be considered. Psychogenic causes of chronic anovulation include anorexia nervosa and amenorrhea of emotional stress; one directs treatment to the primary cause, and estrogen therapy is usually not prescribed if the amenorrhea is short-lived.

Suggested Readings

Bardin CW, Wright W: Androgen receptor deficiency: testicular feminization, its variants, and differential diagnosis. *Ann Clin Res* 12:236, 1980.

Biller BMK, Klibanski A: Amenorrhea and osteoporosis. *Endocrinologist* 1:294, 1991.

Griffin JE, Edwards C, Madden JD, Harrod MJ, Wilson JD: Congenital absence of the vagina. *Ann Intern Med* 85:224, 1976.

Griffin JE, Wilson JD: Disorders of androgen receptor function. *Ann NY Acad Sci* 438:61, 1984.

Klein SM, Garcia CR: Asherman's syndrome: a critique and current review. *Fertil Steril* 24:722, 1973.

Mashchak CA, Kletzky OA, Davajan V: Clinical and laboratory evaluation of patients with primary amenorrhea. *Obstet Gynecol* 57:715, 1981.

Mezrow G, Rebar RW: Tailoring estrogen replacement to fit the patient. *Contemp Ob/Gyn* 31:51, 1988.

Speroff L, Glass RH, Kase NG: Amenorrhea. In *Clinical Gynecologic Endocrinology and Infertility*, ed 4. Baltimore, Williams & Wilkins, 1989, pp 165–211.

Chapter 8

Impotence

Impotence is the inability to achieve or to maintain a penile erection for sexual intercourse. Recurrent or persistent impotence (as opposed to occasional episodes of "honeymoon" impotence) affects some 10 million American men and accounts for at least 400,000 outpatient visits each year. Impotence increases with age, so approximately 20% of the males aged 60 years and 50% of males aged 70 years are impotent.

Libido, the physiological and mental drive for sexual satisfaction, is essential for potency. Libido varies among individuals and within each individual is influenced by social and sexual experiences, by physical and mental illness, and by medication. Libido tends to decrease with age, but loss of sexual interest and drive is most commonly situational. Men may experience dissatisfaction with their accomplishments, frustration, fatigue from overwork, or discouragement and lack of communication with their sexual partner. These factors as well as depression and neurosis account for most impotence in younger men, so-called psychogenic or functional impotence. Drugs that diminish libido include alcohol, tranquilizers, sedatives, opiates, antihypertensives, and estrogens. Hypogonadism affects libido and is discussed below.

Potency also depends on normal anatomy and physiological function. The erectile mechanism requires intact neurological, vascular, and endocrine systems. Impairment of any one of these can produce impotence. The flaccid penis is normally under tonic sympathetic inhibition. This adrenergic discharge results in vasoconstriction of smooth muscle of cavernosal arteries and cavernosal sinusoids. Penile erection begins with central psychogenic stimuli and local sensory stimulation of the genital organs. Stimulation of efferent parasympathetic nerve fibers from the sacral spinal cord to the penis leads to smooth muscle relaxation of cavernosal arteries and sinusoids. The in-

creased blood flow (16 times normal) causes engorgement of the corporal cavernosum. The filling of the corporal cavernosum against the
tunica albuginea causes passive veno-occlusion of outflow that facilitates maintenance of erection. With ejaculation (sympathetic nerve
mediated), arterial smooth muscle tone returns followed by detumes-
cence.

NEUROGENIC IMPOTENCE

Any disruption of the parasympathetic autonomous nervous system
impairs erectile ability. Stimulation of the S2–S4 nerve roots via the
nervi erigentes causes relaxation of specialized vascular smooth muscles. Many diseases interfere with parasympathetic outflow: diabetes
mellitus, alcoholism, heavy metal intoxication, cord tumors, and multiple sclerosis. Surgical procedures such as perineal prostatectomy or
retroperineal dissection also may impair the erectile mechanism.

VASCULAR IMPOTENCE

Full erection requires adequate penile blood flow. Obstruction of the
aorta, iliac vessels, hypogastric, or pudendal arteries can lead to impotence. Leriche's syndrome, an example of vascular impotence, produces lower extremity claudication and impotence. Small arteriole
disease associated with diabetes mellitus also causes impotence. Penile
venous disease shunts cavernosal sinusoidal blood from the normal
veno-occlusion mechanism and leads to a semirigid penis.
Genitourinary conditions such as Peyronie's disease, urethritis, severe
chordee, and penile trauma may result in impotence.

ENDOCRINE IMPOTENCE

The hormone milieu must be adequate for potency. Normal adrenal
and thyroid function are important to male sexual function, but
testosterone production is paramount. Testosterone stimulates protein synthesis (muscle mass) and virilization (enlargement of phallus,
scrotal rugosity and pigmentation, and hair growth on face, chest, and
back). High intratesticular levels of testosterone are essential to normal spermatogenesis. Testosterone also affects the limbic system,
which relates to its effect on libido. Testosterone deficiency (hypogonadism) is an important cause of endocrine impotence and is most
amenable to treatment. The most common cause of organic impotence is diabetes mellitus. This is usually due to a combination of vas-

cular obstruction as a result of arteriosclerosis and autonomic neuropathy.

WORKUP OF IMPOTENT PATIENT
History

The importance of the history cannot be overemphasized. The patient who can sometimes have normal erections and yet be impotent at other times most likely has functional or psychogenic impotence. Normal erections imply that the neurogenic, vascular, and endocrine systems are intact. Ask about early morning penile erections. Interview partner to further clarify factors that contribute to impotence. Does patient have multiple sex partners? Are there identifiable stress factors? If the patient has diabetes mellitus, are there other symptoms of peripheral or autonomic neuropathy? Is there claudication that might explain incomplete penile tumescence? What is the patient's age and when did impotence develop? Failure to virilize by the mid to late teens implies pituitary or gonadal abnormality that must be thoroughly investigated. Are there other endocrine dysfunctions in the past to suggest polyglandular failure? What medications are the patient taking? Common medications associated with impotence include cimetidine, antihypertensives (e.g., propranolol, methyldopa, guanethidine), and antidepressants and antipsychotic medications.

Physical Examination

The physical examination may give clues about hypogonadism. What is testicle size? Normal testes are 4.5 ± 1.0 cm long and 2.5 ± 0.5 cm wide. Are testes pea-sized and firm, typical of Klinefelter's syndrome? Klinefelter's syndrome (primary testicular failure caused by chromatin-positive gonadal dysgenesis), a common cause of hypogonadism, affects 1 of 500 males. Many of these patients develop secondary sex characteristics during puberty because the Leydig's cells have not yet involuted. The skin of the chronic hypogonadal male is smooth and soft with crow's-foot wrinkles about the eyes and mouth. Anosmia suggests hypogonadotropic hypogonadism (Kallman's syndrome). Is there evidence for pituitary disease such as galactorrhea on manual expression of the breast areola to suggest prolactinoma? Physical findings of chronic disease such as hepatic or renal failure and other endocrine diseases such as hypoadrenalism, acromegaly, and hypothyroidism should be sought as potential causes of impotence. Curvature of the flaccid penis may be a cue for Peyronie's disease. In the diabetic with impotence, signs of a concomitant peripheral neuropathy (absent ankle jerks, decreased vibratory sensation) may present. Orthostatic hypotension suggests an underlying autonomic neuropathy.

Laboratory Studies

<u>Serum testosterone</u> should be measured in each impotent patient. Normal adult values range from 270 to 1000 ng/dL. There is some diurnal variation in the serum testosterone; the highest levels occur between 6 and 9 AM with a 15–40% decrement by late afternoon. The lower values are still well within the normal range, so one determination is sufficient for diagnostic purposes. Testosterone production decreases with age, and serum testosterone levels are slightly decreased but remain well within the normal range. Because testosterone production is controlled by luteinizing hormone (LH), any disturbance of the hypothalamic-pituitary-testicular axis may lead to testosterone deficiency and impotency. In primary testicular disease <u>serum LH</u> is very helpful because it is elevated in the absence of the negative feedback of testosterone. Thus, patients with <u>primary hypogonadism</u> have <u>low serum testosterone levels</u> and <u>high serum LH levels</u>.

If serum testosterone and LH levels are low, then pituitary or hypothalamic disease should be investigated. Secondary hypogonadism is often due to a prolactinoma that usually presents late (macroadenoma) with impotence being the predominant clinical symptom. *Serum prolactin* should be ordered if anything suggests hypogonadism in the middle and late age male. A mass lesion may be identified by computed tomography or magnetic resonance imaging. If the serum prolactin is normal and a mass lesion is excluded, then think about hemochromatosis as the cause of the secondary hypogonadism. Occasionally patients with hyperthyroidism present with impotence, but the serum testosterone is elevated (>1200 ng/mL) because hyperthyroidism increases the sex hormone-binding globulin (the free testosterone concentration is normal). Treatment of hyperthyroidism usually corrects the impotence. An occasional diabetic may have primary testicular failure that produces impotence. Because hypogonadism is treatable, one should measure serum testosterone in these patients.

<u>In summary, determination of serum testosterone, serum LH, and serum prolactin usually detects most endocrine causes of impotence.</u>

Etiology of Hypogonadism

Primary hypogonadism may be caused by various disorders. Idiopathic testicular failure, sometimes associated with polyglandular endocrine failure, is the most common. Gonadal dysgenesis, testicular torsion, and trauma are other causes. Secondary hypogonadism may be due to constitutional delay of growth and development in the adolescent, to isolated hypogonadotropic hypogonadism, or to any of the causes of hypopituitarism (page 97). Other endocrine causes such as acromegaly and Addison's disease should be managed before any treatment of associated hypogonadism.

Treatment of Hypogonadism

Testosterone replacement is simple, effective, and safe. Esterified derivatives of testosterone are given intramuscularly, assuring constant levels necessary to maintain muscle mass, beard growth, and libido. Testosterone cypionate or testosterone enanthate 200 mg im every 2–4 weeks restores potency in most hypogonadal males. Replacement is continued indefinitely. Lower doses (50–100 mg im every 2–3 weeks) are used in the adolescent hypogonadal male to avoid excessive stimulation of epiphyseal cartilage growth and maturation. Excessive androgen accelerates the maturation process, leading to bone closure and short stature. Orally administered alkylated testosterone derivatives are *not* used because their effects on potency are not predictable and there are risks of hepatotoxicity with long-term therapy.

Evaluation and Treatment of Nonendocrine Impotence

Evaluation and treatment of the impotent male who is not hypogonadal generally requires referral to a physician or surgeon interested in this problem. Diagnostic injection of the corpora cavernosum with an insulin syringe containing papavarine, phentolamine, or prostaglandin E1 leads to penile engorgement lasting for 2–4 hours in normal men. Failure to erect usually means arterial occlusive disease, although venous disease or sinusoidal scarring is also possible. If a patient is a suitable candidate for revascularization, then referral to a center for diagnostic studies and possible vascular reconstruction (about 10% success rate) is appropriate. If penile tumescence is achieved with vasoactive intracavernosal injection, then pharmacologic erection program (papaverine, phentolamine, or prostaglandin E1) may be implemented. Hazards include priapism, nodules and scarring at site of injection, and possible abnormal liver function studies. However, the safest, cheapest, and also the oldest therapy for impotence uses a <u>vacuum-constriction device</u>. The patient applies a cylinder over the penis, uses a pump that draws blood into the penis by vacuum, and places a rubber or Silastic ring at the base of the penis to impede venous return. Rarely, a mechanical device such as a semi-rigid rod or inflatable prosthesis is advised. Figure 8.1 outlines one approach to evaluate and treat impotence.

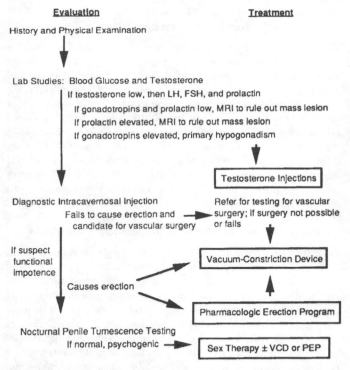

Figure 8.1. Evaluation and treatment of impotence. *FSH*, follicle-stimulating hormone; *MRI*, magnetic resonance imaging; *VCD*, vacuum-constriction device; *PEP*, pharmacologic erection program.

Functional or Psychogenic Impotence

The prevalence of impotence vastly exceeds that of all endocrine disorders. Therefore, most instances of sexual dysfunction are not related to a primary endocrine problem. For patients strongly suspected of a functional cause of impotence, nocturnal penile tumescence study most accurately distinguishes psychogenic from organic impotence. Nocturnal erections are diminished or absent in organic impotence. Androgen treatment of patients with functional impotence is not helpful. Several studies have shown that the effect of testosterone in these patients matches that of placebo therapy alone. Chronic testosterone treatment of eugonadal males decreases sperm count and testicular volume, so this is not even a good placebo drug.

Many men want "just a pill" to help with potency. Some physicians prescribe yohimbine hydrochloride, a drug with α-adrenergic blocking properties, but there is no pill that restores potency. Appropriate evaluation and counseling regarding the pathophysiology of impotence and the factors that affect libido are necessary in treating these patients with psychogenic impotence. These patients may be candidates for vacuum-constriction devices or pharmacologic erection therapy.

Suggested Readings

Krane RJ, Goldstein I, deTejada IS: Impotence. *N Engl J Med* 321:1648, 1989.

Lue TF, Tanagho EA: Physiology of erection and pharmacological management of impotence. *J Urol* 137:829, 1989.

Nadig PW: Evaluating and treating impotence. *Pract Diabetol* 8:1,1989.

Schwartz MF, Kolodny RC, Masters WH: Plasma testosterone levels of sexually functional and dysfunctional men. *Arch Sex Behav* 9:355, 1980.

Spark RF, White RA, Connolly PB: Impotence is not always psychogenic. Newer insights into hypothalamic-pituitary-gonadal dysfunction. *JAMA* 243:750, 1980.

Susset JG, Tessier CD, Wincze J, et al: Effect of yohimbine hydrochloride on erectile impotence: a double blind study. *J Urol* 141:1360, 1989.

Chapter 9

Hirsutism

Women often complain of extra hair and seek advice in managing this cosmetic problem. Hirsutism refers to excessive growth of hair in the androgen-responsive skin zones typically considered to be masculine in distribution. Terminal (coarse) hairs develop on the upper lip, sideburns, chin, neck, chest, lower abdomen (male escutcheon), and perineum. The degree of hair stimulation varies depending on race (Orientals, American Indians, and Negroes have generally less hirsutism than Caucasians), genetic background (those of Mediterranean origin are typically more hirsute than those of Nordic origin), complexion (darkly pigmented Caucasian women tend to be more hirsute than light complected females), age (the incidence of hirsutism increases after menopause), and family history. Although hirsutism may be a marker of underlying disorder, it is not a disease per se. More often than not, hirsutism represents one end of the spectrum of normal hair development. For example, at least 25% of women develop terminal hairs over the lower abdomen, around the areola, and over the upper lip. Each patient interprets hair growth differently. Some women complain of relatively mild hirsutism, not realizing the range of normal variation and the significance of factors mentioned above.

Hyperandrogenism causes hirsutism in most patients (>95%). Testosterone, the primary androgen that stimulates the hair follicle, circulates mostly bound to sex hormone-binding globulin (SHBG); a small fraction (1–3%) circulates as free or unbound testosterone. Nearly all hirsute women have an increased testosterone production rate, although the serum or plasma testosterone may be in the upper range of normal. Three sources produce testosterone in the normal female: ovary (25% of total), adrenal (25% of total), and peripheral tissues (50% of total). The peripheral tissues (fat, muscle) convert weak androgens (primarily androstenedione) secreted by the adrenal and ovary into testosterone. Hair growth in androgen-sensitive areas results from the metabolism of androgens locally at the hair follicle. Increased circulating levels of free testosterone lead to binding of testosterone with androgen receptors at follicles of thin vellus hair. The testosterone-receptor interaction stimulates 5-α-reductase, which converts testosterone to dihydrotestosterone, a very potent androgen responsible for proliferation and growth of thick terminal hair. Once 5-α-reductase is induced by testosterone, other less potent androgens (such as dihydroepiandrosterone (DHEA) and androstenedione) may serve as substrates for the enzyme, leading to dihydrotestosterone formation. This system allows for a multiplier effect, in that weaker androgens now become potent steroids because they lead to local production of dihydrotestosterone within the hair follicle. The metabolism of testosterone at the hair follicle may be associated with a fall of serum testosterone levels despite continued hair growth. Hyperandrogenemia lowers SHBG levels (decreases hepatic SHBG production) so that the total serum testosterone may not accurately reflect the androgen status. Table 9.1 lists the causes of androgen-dependent hirsutism.

Table 9.1
Causes of Androgen-Dependent Hirsutism

Ovarian
    Virilizing ovarian tumors (hilar cell, arrhenoblastoma)
    Severe insulin resistance

Adrenal
    Virilizing adrenal tumors (adrenal adenoma or carcinoma)
    Cushing's disease
    Ectopic adrenocorticotropin-secreting tumors
    Congenital adrenal hyperplasia
        21-hydroxylase deficiency
        3-β-hydroxysteroid dehydrogenase deficiency
        11-hydroxylase deficiency

Combined ovary and adrenal causes
    PCOS (mostly ovary source)
    Idiopathic hirsutism

WORKUP

The evaluation of the hirsute woman need not be complicated. History and physical examination along with judicious laboratory testing indicate the underlying disorder.

History

Facts regarding age and mode of onset of hair growth, menstrual abnormalities, medications, and family history should be sought.

Age of Onset

Was it before the onset of menstruation? Was pubic and axillary hair growth associated with hirsutism? (Hirsutism before age 9 suggests an adrenal source such as congenital adrenal hyperplasia.) Did hair growth start soon after menarche? Progress slowly since menarche? (If yes, then history is typical of either polycystic ovary syndrome (PCOS) or idiopathic hirsutism.) Did hirsutism start at menopause or later? (If it starts several years after menopause, beware of an androgen-secreting tumor of the ovary or the adrenal gland.)

Mode of Onset

Did hirsutism develop gradually or have an abrupt onset? (Abrupt or recent onset suggests significant pathology, i.e., an androgen-secreting tumor.)

Menstrual Abnormalities

Are menses regular? If so, then significant ovary or adrenal pathology is unlikely. Menstrual abnormalities with chronic anovulation are the rule in severe PCOS. Although hirsutism is rare in hyperprolactinemic states, a history of galactorrhea should be sought.

Medications

Is the patient taking drugs that are known to promote hirsutism? Androgens, phenytoin, diazoxide, and minoxidil are known to do this to varying degrees.

Family History

Is there a family history of chronic ovulatory problems? Any wedge resections of ovaries for PCOS? PCOS appears to be inherited as an autosomal dominant trait, and the family history is positive in 40% of cases with PCOS.

Examination

Physical examination should tell whether the patient is simply hirsute or whether virilization is present. The virilized patient is not only severely hirsute but also has clitoromegaly, frontal or occipital balding, deepening of voice, enlargement of thyroid cartilage (Adam's apple), and increased muscle mass. Breast atrophy and loss of body contours occur with severe virilization. Virilization outside the neonatal period suggests a tumor of the ovary or adrenal, although severe PCOS may sometimes cause virilization. Physical stigmata of Cushing's syndrome should be sought. The pelvic examination is particularly important in assessing perineal hair distribution, clitoromegaly, uterus, and adnexal masses. Obese females may need ultrasonography to determine ovary size.

Laboratory

Laboratory studies to identify underlying disorders include serum testosterone, serum 17-hydroxyprogesterone (OHP), serum prolactin, and serum gonadotropins (follicle-stimulating hormone (FSH) and luteinizing hormone (LH)). The most important is serum <u>testosterone</u>. Most women's total serum testosterone is <40 ng/dL, although normal levels can range up to 60 ng/dL. Values above 200 ng/dL indicate significant pathology such as ovary or adrenal tumor, but such levels may be seen in PCOS and in insulin resistance. Free testosterone levels are also generally elevated in hirsute women. It offers no advantage except the patient who has high normal to modestly elevated serum testosterone who may have proportionally higher free testosterone levels to explain the hirsutism. <u>17-OHP</u> screens for 17-hydroxylase deficiency, the most common cause of congenital adrenal hyperplasia. An elevated <u>serum FSH</u> indicates primary ovary failure that might be found in an amenorrheic hirsute patient. <u>Serum LH</u> may be elevated in PCOS or ovary failure, but a normal LH does not eliminate PCOS. <u>Serum prolactin</u> assesses hyperprolactinemia by looking for a prolactinoma in an amenorrheic female; however, elevated prolactins do not cause hirsutism. Serum <u>dehydro-3-epiandosterone sulfate (DHEA-S)</u> is often mildly elevated in hirsute women, although values above 700 mg/dL suggest an adrenal cause. Urine 17-ketosteroids reflect the serum DHEA-S concentrations but do not measure testosterone and are rarely sufficient to evaluate hyperandrogenic syndromes. If Cushing's syndrome cannot be excluded clinically, order a 24-hour urine cortisol or an overnight dexamethasone study (page 14). Androstanediol glucuronide, the androgen metabolite originally proposed as a sensitive marker of hirsutism, is not generally available. Furthermore, recent data suggest it is a marker of adrenal androgen secretion rather than peripheral androgen action. Dynamic studies such as dexamethasone suppression studies and gonadotropin stimulatory studies do *not* help distinguish whether the androgen source is the adrenal or ovary, and they are best avoided.

The source of the hyperandrogenemia can often be identified on the basis of the history, physical examination, and these laboratory studies. Drug-related hirsutism is diagnosed by the history. Therapy can be directed to the specific cause of the hirsutism.

Virilizing Tumors

Androgen-secreting tumors are associated with serum testosterone of >200 ng/dL or DHEA-S >700 μg/dL, rapidly progressing hirsutism with virilization, and an onset usually much later than menarche. The ovary is the usual site of testosterone-producing tumors (arrhenoblastoma, Sertoli-Leydig's cell tumor, etc.), and the adrenal is the site of carcinomas that produce excessive amounts of DHEA-S and urinary 17-ketosteroids. Localization of the androgen-secreting tumor with computed tomography is recommended because an occasional adrenal tumor may secrete only testosterone and be missed if surgery is prematurely directed to the ovaries. After surgery the patient should not expect much reduction in terminal hair; only the rate of growth and hair shaft thickness decrease, causing frustration in the uninformed patient.

Polycystic Ovary Syndrome

Most women who present with hirsutism do not have any ominous cause but rather fit into a spectrum of syndromes associated with normal or modestly elevated serum testosterone and elevated free testosterone. Most are associated with varying degrees of ovary stromal hyperplasia. PCOS is by far the most common variant. PCOS has its onset just after menarche. It is characterized by chronic anovulation (amenorrhea/oligomenorrhea and dysfunctional uterine bleeding) and slowly progressive hirsutism. A familial tendency may be noted for similar problems. Many patients are obese. Some women have no hirsutism but present for evaluation of infertility. Enlarged ovaries are palpable in about half the subjects. The ratio of LH to FSH is often elevated (>2.5).

There is a self-perpetuating cycle of hormone events associated with polycystic ovaries. Increased ovarian production of testosterone blocks follicular maturation, leading to numerous follicles in varying stages of development. These follicles have limited growth potential and undergo atresia, leading to an increase in the stromal compartment. The stroma normally secretes significant amounts of testosterone and androstenedione, and its increased mass results in secretion of a greater amount of androgen. Peripheral conversion of androstenedione into estrone sensitizes the pituitary gonadotrope (as normally happens with increased estrogen levels before the midcycle LH surge) to respond to gonadotropin-releasing hormone, leading to LH production. Estrone also negatively feeds back on FSH production, causing an increased LH:FSH ratio. LH stimulates the ovarian stroma to produce more testosterone (which stimulates hair growth and blocks ovarian follicular maturation, leading to atresia, etc.) and androstenedione (which is converted to estrone and leads to more LH production, etc.). What triggers the cycle is unknown, possibly a hypothalamic defect in gonadotropin-releasing hormone-LH regulation.

Treatment of PCOS is directed toward suppression of ovary production of androgens using oral contraceptive agents. Ortho-Novum 2 mg and Demulen have had wide use for treating PCOS. Ortho-Novum 2 mg is started on the 5th day of menses and is given for 21 days and repeated cyclically. After 2–3 months of treatment, androgen levels are remeasured. If these results are normal or if there has been >50% reduction, treatment is continued, realizing that any amelioration of the hirsutism will be gradual with a maximal therapeutic effect after 9–12 months. The usual precautions related to oral contraceptives (blood pressure, venous thrombosis, etc.) are necessary. Weight reduction should be encouraged if the patient is overweight. Clomiphene may be used to induce ovulation in those patients who desire pregnancy. Ovary wedge resection reduces the stromal compartment and may benefit patients who fail to ovulate with clomiphene. Pulsatile gonadotropin-releasing hormone has also been used in patients who desire pregnancy and who fail with clomiphene.

If there is galactorrhea/hyperprolactinemia, the hyperandrogenism is part of the amenorrhea-galactorrhea syndrome associated with PCOS and overproduction of adrenal androgens. The mechanism of hyperandrogenism in this syndrome is not understood. Treatment of the hyperprolactinemia with bromocriptine (or surgical removal of the prolactinoma) may help the hirsutism.

Late-Onset Congenital Adrenal Hyperplasia

A few hirsute females (often with normal menstruation and very mild hair growth) have a late-onset or adult form of congenital adrenal hyperplasia. In this syndrome, there is a partial block in 21-hydroxylase activity that leads to elevated serum levels of 17-OHP. The diagnosis of attenuated 21-hydroxylase deficiency (late-onset variant of congenital adrenal hyperplasia) must be made biochemically since it is clinically indistinguishable from simple hirsutism or PCOS. Elevated serum 17-OHP levels define the disorder. Normal women have serum 17-OHP below 2 ng/mL in the morning during 1st week after menses; in fact, the mean is usually <1 ng/mL. Slightly higher levels (up to 2.5 ng/mL) occur in the luteal phase of the menstrual cycle. With adrenocorticotropin stimulation (cosyntropin 0.25 mg iv or im), 17-OHP levels obtained 30–60 minutes later rarely rise above 3.5 ng/mL in normal women. In the homozygous form of this disorder, basal or nonstimulated 17-OHP levels are >10 ng/mL. Clinically, this is not a diagnostic problem because the disorder usually manifests in infant females with ambiguous genitalia. However, for unknown reasons the attenuated variety of 21-hydroxylase deficiency may present with hirsutism years later. Mildly elevated 17-OHP between 2 and 10 ng/mg can be seen in both homozygous and heterozygous 21-hydroxylase deficiency (the latter is not associated with hirsutism) as well as in PCOS. Adrenocorticotropin stimulation distinguishes these conditions; 17-OHP rises above 10 ng/dL in homozygous 21-hydroxylase deficiency. Patients who stimulate from 0.1 to 1.6 ng/mL may have a 16-fold rise, but the criteria for diagnosis rests on the absolute magnitude. Figure 9.1 helps screen for these disorders.

The true incidence of attenuated 17-hydroxylase deficiency is unknown, ranging from 0 of 38 hirsute women to 5 of 25 hirsute women. The author's experience reflects that of Chetkowski et al. in which this disorder accounts for about 1% of hirsute women. The message is "attenuated 21-hydroxylase is a rare cause of hirsutism." Be very reticent to place hirsute women on glucocorticoids unless congenital adrenal

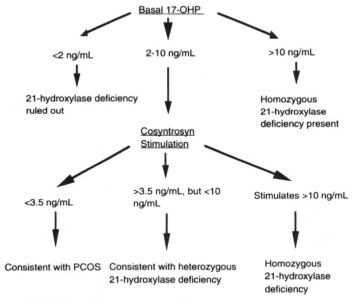

Figure 9.1. Flow diagram to screen for 21-hydroxylase deficiency.

hyperplasia is confirmed. Prednisone, for example, is difficult to adjust and monitor, and the associated weight gain is a "no-no" for them. It is best to make sure the criteria are well established before submitting adult females to this form of therapy. Finally, making the diagnosis may be intellectually rewarding, but practically speaking these hirsute women appear to respond to antiandrogen, such as spironolactone, as well as to glucocorticoids.

Idiopathic Hirsutism

Some hirsute females have normal menses and normal serum androgens. These women have idiopathic hirsutism probably caused by increased sensitivity of the hair follicle to normal circulating amounts of androgens. Treatment with spironolactone generally helps these patients. Some physicians prefer oral contraceptives because serum testosterone falls with ovary suppression. In addition, since estrogens increase SHBG, the level of free testosterone is lower. The antiandrogen drug, cyproterone acetate, appears to be the most effective medication for idiopathic hirsutism but is not approved for use in the United States.

TREATMENT

Most women have a benign form of hirsutism that requires attention and sympathy. Mechanical methods (bleaching, shaving, plucking, waxing, and depilatory creams) work well with very mild hirsutism. In these patients, such treatments produce cosmetically acceptable results. Shaving is the easiest, safest, and least expensive method to remove visible hairs. Patients should be informed that shaving does *not* increase hair growth or increase the thickness of the hair shaft. The only permanent means of removing the hair is to ablate the hair follicle, generally by electrolysis. Electrolysis or short-wave radio frequency thermolysis coagulates the hair root and requires the skill of an experienced electrologist. Electrolysis is time-consuming and expensive, may be painful, and is best used for few terminal hairs or in combination with medical therapy.

Medical therapy can offer help but is notoriously unsatisfactory for many patients. Hirsutism, although not a disease, can be perceived as an ugly, unattractive blight (particularly in teenage years) or a nuisance requiring shaving once or twice a day. The physician must discern among the possible benefits versus side effects, cost, and complications of drugs. Drug treatment attempts to suppress ovary or adrenal androgen production or to block androgen action with antiandrogens (androgen receptor blockers). Medical therapy usually halts the progression of new hair development, slows hair growth, and sometimes causes hair regression, particularly vellus hair. Patients with mild hirsutism and regular menses respond to antiandrogens such as spironolactone 25–50 mg bid. The major side effect is increased menstrual frequency in 10–20% of women. Hirsute patients with oligomenorrhea/amenorrhea do well with oral contraceptives ± spironolactone. Cyproterone acetate, the most prescribed antiandrogen in Europe, is not available in the United States. Flutamide, another antiandrogen, is too costly (six times spironolactone) and is approved only for prostatic carcinoma in the United States. Gonadotropin-releasing factor analogs provide great ovary suppression but are quite expensive and impractical. Drugs only control and rarely cure, and they must be continued indefinitely, another factor that patients should know about medical therapy. Patients should be informed that months of therapy are necessary before calling a medication ineffective. Do not promise too much, and be realistic about the expectations of medical treatment. The combination of frequent shaving, judicious electrolysis, medical therapy, and a sympathetic physician is necessary to successfully manage this common medical problem.

Suggested Readings

Barth JH, Cherry CA, Wojnarowska F, Dawber RPR: Cyproterone acetate for severe hirsutism: results of a double-blind dose-ranging study. *Clin Endocrinol* (Oxf) 35:5, 1991.

Burch WM: Commentary: a women with too much facial hair. *N C Med J* 53:521,1992.

Chetkowski RJ, DeFazio J, Shamonki I, et al: The incidence of late-onset congenital adrenal hyperplasia due to 21-hydroxylase deficiency among hirsute women. *J Clin Endocrinol Metab* 58:595, 1984.

Dunaif A: Insulin resistance and ovarian hyperandrogenism. *Endocrinologist* 2:248, 1992.

Givens JR: Hirsutism. In Krieger DT, Bardin CW (eds): *Current Therapy in Endocrinology 1983–1984*. Burlington, Ontario, Decker, 1983, pp 143–146.

Kirschner MA, Zucker IR, Jepersen D: Idiopathic hirsutism—anovarian abnormality. *N Engl J Med* 294:637, 1976.

Kuttenn F, Couillin P, Girard F, et al: Late-onset adrenal hyperplasia. *N Engl J Med* 313:224, 1985.

Lobo R, Horton R: Hirsutism. In Krieger DT, Bardin CW (eds): *Current Therapy in Endocrinology 1985–1986*. Burlington, Ontario, Decker, 1985, pp 131–134.

Pehrson JJ, Vaitukaitis J, Longcope C: Bromocriptine, sex steroid metabolism, and menstrual patterns in the polycystic ovarian syndrome. *Ann Intern Med* 105:129, 1986.

Rittmaster RS, Loriaux DL: Hirsutism. *Ann Intern Med* 106:95, 1987.

Rittmaster RS: Treating hirsutism. *Endocrinologist* 3: 211, 1993.

Yen SSC: The polycystic ovary syndrome. *Clin Endocrinol* 12:177, 1980.

Zumoff B, Freeman R, Coupey S, et al: A chronobiologic abnormality in luteinizing hormone secretion in teenage girls with the polycystic-ovary syndrome. *N Engl J Med* 309:1206, 1983.

Chapter 10

Gynecomastia

Gynecomastia (male breast hypertrophy) is a frequent finding because most males have breast enlargement sometime during their life. Small amounts of gynecomastia are common: up to 30% of normal young men have palpable breast tissue; the prevalence increases to 50% in normal older men and 70% of elderly, hospitalized men. Breast development is the same for males and females until puberty when estrogen levels rise dramatically in females. <u>Estrogen</u> is the primary hormone that stimulates both ductal and stromal breast development. Estradiol, a potent estrogen, stimulates breast enlargement in both sexes. Aromatization of testosterone's A ring accounts for most of the estradiol produced in men and occurs primarily in fat tissue. About 10% of serum estradiol comes from its direct secretion from the testes. The fraction of testicular estradiol secretion increases upon gonadotropin (luteinizing hormone (LH)) administration. Estrone is another estrogen produced by the peripheral aromatization of androstenedione, an androgen secreted primarily by the adrenal. The levels of estrogen circulating in the adult male are about 200–300 times lower than serum testosterone levels, yet a perturbation of the ratio of androgen to estrogen by increased estrogen production or decreased testosterone production explains most causes of gynecomastia.

Gynecomastia may be a <u>normal physiological event</u>, <u>a response to drugs and medications</u>, or <u>a harbinger of disease</u>. Gynecomastia can be unilateral and have no other explanation (other than the causes of bilateral breast development). However, care must be taken not to miss the unusual lesions such as breast carcinoma, neurofibroma, hemangioma, and lipoma that all have a different texture on palpation than the finely nodular texture of glandular breast tissue.

GYNECOMASTIA AS A PHYSIOLOGICAL EVENT

There are three stages of life (neonatal, pubertal, and senescent) during which gynecomastia relates to normal development. Neonatal gynecomastia is a transient phenomenon, occurs in response to maternal estrogens, and resolves usually within a few weeks of birth. Pubertal gynecomastia occurs in up to 70% of boys and is probably related to increased testicular production of estradiol. Levels of estradiol peak before adult levels of testosterone are obtained, leading to a temporary alteration of the androgen-to-estrogen ratio. In most boys pubertal gynecomastia disappears within 2–3 years. Large amounts of breast tissue, described as Tanner stage III or greater (glandular tissue that extends past the areola associated with enlargement and darkening of the areola), that persist beyond the age of 16–17 years seldom regress. These young men with persistent pubertal gynecomastia require surgical removal of the glandular tissue. Senescent gynecomastia found in the seventh and eighth decades of life is a diagnosis of exclusion since there are many causes of gynecomastia (e.g., drugs or underlying disease) in this age group. Slightly decreased testosterone levels and increased peripheral aromatization of testosterone to estradiol produce an altered androgen-to-estrogen ratio that causes the gynecomastia in these men.

GYNECOMASTIA RELATED TO DRUG USE

Drugs cause gynecomastia by many mechanisms. Inhibitors of testosterone synthesis include ketoconazole and chemotherapeutic drugs (cyclophosphamide, melphalan, etc.). Cimetidine and spironolactone inhibit testosterone action at the receptor level. Any medication that increases the levels of estrogen or its effect may lead to gynecomastia. Testosterone therapy itself can cause gynecomastia by peripheral conversion to estradiol. Digitalis and digitoxin are weak estrogen agonists. Diethylstilbestrol therapy used to treat prostatic carcinoma causes gynecomastia that can be prevented with pretreatment irradiation to the breasts (900–1500 rad over 3 days). Treatment with human chorionic gonadotropin (HCG) increases testicular production of estrogens. Other anecdotal associations of drug-related gynecomastia include digoxin, methyldopa, reserpine, isoniazid, ethionamide, tricyclic antidepressants, phenothiazines, diazepam, hydroxyzine, heroin, and marijuana.

GYNECOMASTIA RELATED TO UNDERLYING DISORDER OR DISEASE

Hypogonadism as a result of decreased testosterone production or a decrease in its action may cause gynecomastia. Primary testicular failure related to Klinefelter's syndrome (incidence of about 0.2% in the male population) is common and is frequently associated with gynecomastia. Other causes of testicular failure (e.g., anorchism, trauma, orchitis) may be associated with gynecomastia. Gynecomastia found in androgen resistance syndromes such as perineoscrotal hypospadias (Reifenstein's syndrome) is caused by testosterone's decreased effect on typically androgen-sensitive tissues and by increased LH stimulation of testicular estradiol secretion, leading to an altered ratio of effective androgen to estrogen.

Increased estrogen production caused by feminizing tumors of the adrenal gland and Leydig's cell tumors of the testes is rare. The production of estrogen can be a direct release of estradiol from the tumor or, as in the case of adrenal tumors, an increase in precursor substrate concentration (androstenedione) that is converted to estrogen peripherally. Tumors most likely to cause gynecomastia are gonadotropin-secreting tumors such as oat cell lung carcinoma, choriocarcinoma, and hepatoblastoma. Testicular aromatase activity is enhanced by HCG, leading to increased estradiol secretion.

Certain metabolic and chronic diseases are associated with gynecomastia. Increased substrate for the aromatase enzyme is a common cause of raised estrogen levels. Hyperthyroidism is associated with increased production of adrenal steroids including androstenedione, leading to peripheral estrone production and gynecomastia. Also, sex hormone-binding globulin levels are increased in hyperthyroidism. This leads to elevated total serum testosterone and estradiol levels. Because estradiol binds less avidly to sex hormone-binding globulin than testosterone, free estradiol is elevated while free testosterone is normal in hyperthyroid patients. The metabolism and removal of androstenedione are impaired in chronic liver disease, again leading to increased substrate for the aromatase enzyme. Hyperprolactinemia per se does not cause gynecomastia, but an elevated prolactin inhibts LH release, leading to lower serum testosterone levels that change the androgen-to-estrogen ratio. Refeeding gynecomastia occurs in debilitated patients recovering from starvation and serious systemic illness such as uremia (dialysis) and heart failure.

WORKUP

The history and physical examination identify most causes of gynecomastia. The recent onset of breast enlargement deserves particular attention. Age of the patient is important as it relates to physiological causes of gynecomastia. Is there history of recovery from serious illness and malnutrition? Has the patient started dialysis? A history of impotence suggests hypogonadism. Highlight any drug and medication history. Gynecomastia should be worked up if the drug history is negative, if the breast is tender (possibly reflecting rapid growth), if breast mass is >4 cm, or if clinical state dictates further evaluation (e.g., hypogonadism).

The physical examination should be complete and focus on the breast, testes, and liver. In the obese male one often has difficulty distinguishing adipose tissue (lipomastia) from glandular tissue. A good method to determine whether breast tissue is present is to place the pulp of the index finger directly over the nipple and apply pressure. One encounters no resistance and easily palpates the underlying rib and intercostal space in the normal and obese male. This area is obscured by glandular tissue in patients with gynecomastia. True gynecomastia can be distinguished from lipomastia by mammography or sonography. If there is unilateral breast enlargement, one should take care to examine for signs of cancer (firmness and fixation to skin and surrounding fascia as well as enlarged axillary nodes). Gynecomastia does not predispose the male breast to carcinoma except in men with Klinefelter's syndrome (the mechanism for the 10- to 20-fold increase is unknown). The testes are examined for masses. Testicular size and consistency should be recorded. Leydig's cell tumors can be small and may require ultrasound if there is significant hyperestrogenemia. Is there hepatomegaly? Are there skin signs of hyperestrogenism (e.g., spider angioma)? Is there a goiter or tachycardia to suggest hyperthyroidism? Figure 10.1 diagrams an approach to evaluate gynecomastia.

LABORATORY

The laboratory studies ordered are cued from the history and physical examination. Liver function is assessed by checking the transaminases, alkaline phosphatase, and bilirubin. The adolescent male with persistent pubertal gynecomastia rarely needs any studies if there is good health, normal growth and development, and a normal genital

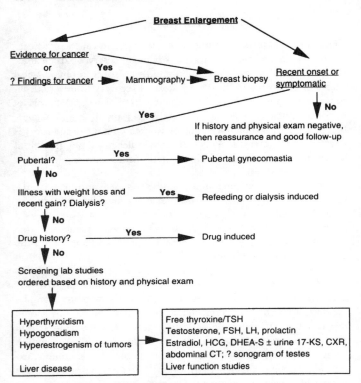

Figure 10.1. Flow diagram to evaluate gynecomastia. *TSH,* thyroid-stimulating hormone; *FSH,* follicle-stimulating hormone; *DHEA-S,* dehydroepiandrosterone-sulfate; *KS,* ketosteroid; *CXR,* chest X-ray; *CT,* computed tomography.

examination. <u>Klinefelter's syndrome</u> (small firm testes) should be confirmed by leukocyte chromosomal karotyping (or a buccal smear looking for sex chromatin XXY). Serum determinations of testosterone, LH, and prolactin are obtained particularly when there is a history of impotence. If the LH is high and testosterone is low, then the diagnosis is primary testicular failure. If both LH and testosterone are low in a patient with gynecomastia, then the diagnosis most likely is increased estrogen production (e.g., Sertoli's cell tumor of testes). If both LH and testosterone are elevated, the diagnosis is either androgen resistance state or gonadotropin-secreting tumor. Sertun HCG (not urine for pregnancy test) and chest X-ray are necessary to exclude tumor-related gynecomastia. Other endocrine studies include serum thyroid-stimulating hormone to exclude hyperthyroidism and serum dehydroepiandrosterone-sulfate or urinary 17-ketosteroids to exclude a feminizing adrenal tumor (these are rare and bulky tumors easily identified on abdominal computed tomography). Even with measurement of serum estradiol and these other studies, the cause of the gynecomastia may not be found, probably reflecting the "normalcy" of this state.

TREATMENT

Management of gynecomastia depends on its cause. Patients who have suspicious findings for breast carcinoma need biopsy. For those men with an equivocal examination or large breasts, order a mammogram. Discontinuation of the offending medication is often associated with regression of minor degrees of gynecomastia. Large amounts of breast tissue rarely regress even after the cause is removed. Reduction mammoplasty is the only effective therapy for these patients. Young men with persistent pubertal gynecomastia need surgical excision since the personal and psychological problems these males encounter are real, and cosmetic reduction preserving the areola is beneficial.

Suggested Readings

Brody SA, Loriaux DL: Gynecomastia. In Krieger DT, Bardin CW (eds); *Current Therapy in Endocrinology 1985–1986*. Burlington, Ontario, Decker, 1985, pp 185–187.

Carlson HE: Gynecomastia: pathogenesis and therapy. *Endocrinologist* 1:337, 1991.

Korenman SG: The endocrinology of the abnormal male breast. *Ann NY Acad Sci* 464:400, 1986.

Niewoehner CG, Nuttall FQ: Gynecomastia in a hospitalized male population. *Am J Med* 77:633, 1984.

Nuttall FQ: Gynecomastia as a physical finding in normal men. *J Clin Endocrinol Metab* 48:338, 1979.

Wilson JD, Aiman J, MacDonald PC: The pathogenesis of gynecomastia. *Adv Intern Med* 25:1, 1980.

Chapter 11

Thyroid Disease

THYROID NODULES

The nodular thyroid gland is a common and important clinical problem found in up to 5% of the adult female population. Public awareness that nodules are associated with cancer has heightened the anxiety related to this diagnosis, yet the number of annual new cases of thyroid cancer is only 0.004% (39/million). Therein lies the difficulty. The risk is real, but the chances are small that any given patient has thyroid cancer. To remove every nodular thyroid would submit numerous patients to surgery, most of whom have a benign and mostly asymptomatic disorder. Fortunately, it is possible to identify factors which increase the likelihood that a nodule represents cancer of the thyroid. These risk factors are age, sex, history of irradiation, history of familial thyroid carcinoma, and certain physical characteristics of the thyroid itself.

Age

Thyroid nodules are rare in children, but about half of them are malignant. There is often a history of radiation exposure. Therefore nodules found in patients younger than 16 years should be excised.

Sex

Thyroid nodules are five times more common in females than males. Thyroid cancer is also more frequent in females, but only by a factor of two. Therefore there is a greater risk of cancer in a male with a thyroid nodule than in a female who has a thyroid nodule.

History of Irradiation

Irradiation of the head and neck (50–700 rad) increases the risk of thyroid cancer. The period of latency ranges from 5 to 35 years with the average around 20 years after exposure. Nodules should be removed in patients with this history.

History of Familial Thyroid Carcinoma

Medullary thyroid carcinoma (sometimes associated with hyperparathyroidism and pheochromocytoma as multiple endocrine adenomatosis type II) is often familial (20% of the cases). A history for this should be sought. A positive family history is an indication for a plasma calcitonin; an elevated value confirms the diagnosis.

Physical Characteristics of Thyroid Gland

The single nodule is much more likely to be malignant than the multinodular gland. The recent onset of a rapidly enlarging, firm neck mass (especially with associated hoarseness) is suggestive of infiltrative malignant disease. A thyroid mass presenting as a single palpable nodule (or as part of a multinodular gland) that is very firm, irregular, or adherent to overlying muscle generally needs surgical excision. Carcinomatous thyroid cells do not trap radionuclides as well as normal thyroid cells, leading to hypofunctioning, "cold areas" on thyroid scan. Hyperfunctioning or "hot" nodules on radionuclide iodine scans are very, very unlikely to be malignant. However, even most cold nodules are *not* malignant; thus hypofunction of the nodule is not itself very helpful in making the decision to recommend surgery. Cysts of the thyroid represent approximately 10–15% of cold thyroid nodules. These can be identified by ultrasound studies. Simple cysts are rarely malignant and can be treated with aspiration. Cyst fluid should be sent for cytologic examination because cystic degeneration within large neoplastic lesions occurs. Positive or suspicious cytology requires surgical removal of the cyst.

Although these factors help to select high risk patients, only examination of tissue from the nodule is definite. In this regard fine needle aspiration helps immensely in the diagnosis and management of the solitary thyroid nodule. The critical, absolutely essential factor in

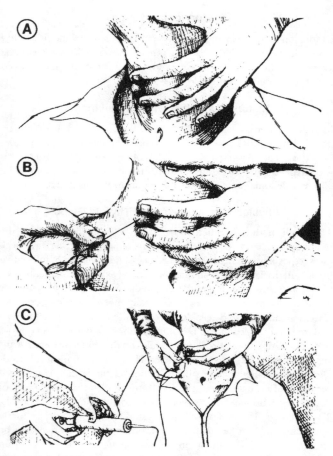

Figure 11.1.   Method of fine needle aspiration biopsy. **A,** patient is seated in a chair, and nodule is localized. **B,** needle is inserted into nodule. **C,** assistant aspirates syringe.

needle aspiration is the availability of a cytopathologist who is expert in interpreting thyroid pathology. Fine needle aspiration offers a rational approach to managing the thyroid nodule. Furthermore, it is safe and the most cost effective method to evaluate the nodular thyroid. Because the thyroid is best palpated with the patient sitting or standing, I use the following technique of needle aspiration since small nodules can be well-localized and fixed between the fingers to allow adequate sampling of thyroid tissue.

The physician stands behind the patient who sits upright in a chair. The area over the nodule is prepared with a local antiseptic. No anesthetic is used. The nodule is fixed between the index and third finger. Having the patient swallow water helps center the nodule between these fingers as demonstrated in Figure 11.1A. A 21- to 23-gauge needle is affixed to a plastic connecting tube (Venotube, Abbott Labs). The hub of the needle is held between the thumb and index finger of the other hand (Fig. 11.1B). The needle is quickly inserted into the mass. The needle may be twirled to enhance movement of cells into the bore of the needle. Once a small drop of material is seen at the top of the needle, the needle is removed. If fluid is encountered, an assistant attaches a syringe and aspirates the syringe's obturator (Fig. 11.1C).

The nodule can be massaged as the fluid is being aspirated. Any fluid is sent for cytology in a heparinized tube (green stoppered Vacutainer works well) on ice. Any scant material is forced by air onto a glass slide and fixed as any other cytologic material (70–90% ethanol works well— some cytopathologists like air-dried slides as well). Alternatively, one can modify this "nonaspirating" technique by attaching a syringe to the connecting tube and having an assistant pull the syringe's obturator. Make sure the syringe is disconnected before removing the needle from the nodule to avoid aspirating material into the tubing. Avoid aspirating only the center of a large nodule, which may yield degenerated, necrotic material. Multiple passes can be made to assure adequacy of the sample. The needle may be washed free of cells with normal saline into a heparinized tube and sent to cytopathology on ice. There the cells can be washed with increasing concentrations of ethanol, which lyses red blood cells, filtered through a

Millipore filter, and then stained for interpretation by the cytopathologist.

WORKUP AND MANAGEMENT OF THYROID NODULE

The following should be performed in all patients with thyroid nodule(s): (*a*) history and physical examination with special attention to palpating the neck for lymph nodes and the physical characteristics of the thyroid gland; (*b*) thyroid function studies including thyroid-stimulating hormone (TSH); and (*c*) if there is clinical evidence of malignancy such as a child with a single firm thyroid nodule or if there is a history of radiation exposure, surgical removal is recommended. Otherwise, <u>fine needle aspiration is routinely performed</u>.

If the aspiration cytology is suspicious or positive for malignancy, then surgery is recommended. If the cytologic diagnosis is <u>follicular neoplasm</u>, surgery is also advised since the cytopathologist cannot differentiate follicular adenoma from follicular carcinoma. Management for all other cytologic diagnoses (e.g., colloid nodule, hemorrhagic cyst, etc.) depends on the functional characteristics of the nodule. If a nondiagnostic or unsatisfactory specimen is obtained (not enough cells for the cytopathologist to make a call), then reaspirate. One may be reasonably sure of the benign nature of a thyroid lesion in the following circumstances. (*a*) The sudden development of a thyroid nodule associated with pain for 4–5 days; this usually represents hemorrhage into a cyst or adenoma. Aspiration confirms the diagnosis. (*b*) Very high titers of antimicrosomal antibodies and needle aspiration biopsy are compatible with a nodular form of Hashimoto's thyroiditis. TSH may or may not be elevated. (*c*) Multinodular goiter with patchy uptake on thyroid scan; if there is an area of unusual firmness, fine needle aspiration is performed. (*d*) The nodule is hot on scan, and the rest of the gland is suppressed. Thyroid scintiscan often is obtained where there is no cytopathologist experienced in reading thyroid aspirates and in patients who are treated with thyroid for thyroid suppression and have increased serum levels of thyroxine (T4). Here the scintiscan and thyroid uptake are obtained to determine if the mass is functioning. A single hot nodule on technetium scan does not rule out malignancy, but a similar pattern on 123-iodine or 131-iodine rarely, if ever, is cancer.

Most nodules of the thyroid, including thyroid carcinoma, are responsive to TSH. Traditionally, exogenous thyroid is prescribed with the goal of reducing endogenous TSH secretion yet maintaining the euthyroid status of these patients by treatment with L-thyroxine 0.1–0.2 mg/day. The dose is determined by assessing the serum TSH after 1 month of therapy to ensure that TSH is at or just below lower limits of normal (suggestive range 0.2–0.4 μU/mL) but not in the hyperthyroid range (<0.1 μU/mL). Thyroid suppression is continued for 6–12 months. **If any thyroid nodule grows in the face of adequate thyroid suppression (except for hemorrhage into a cyst or adenoma), it is a strong indication to remove the thyroid nodule.** If there is more than a 50% decrease in the thyroid nodule or the nodule disappears, thyroid suppression is continued indefinitely. If there has been less than a 50% decrease in size, the nodule is reaspirated to see if the original findings can be reproduced. If the cytology is suspicious or is consistent with malignancy, surgical removal is indicated. If both the cytology and nodule size are unchanged after an adequate period of suppression (i.e., 1 year), I favor discontinuing the T4. This avoids keeping patients on a lifelong regimen that does not work (i.e., reduce nodule size). Because there are 2–3% false-negative results with fine needle aspiration, good follow-up is a necessity.

Checking the serum levels of T4 after 1 month of therapy also ensures that the patient (e.g., one with multinodular goiter) has not become hyperthyroid because of autonomous or nonsuppressible nodules. In such a patient with a nonsuppressible nodule on L-thyroxine treatment, the 24-hour 131-iodine uptake is above 5% and the nodule(s) is evident on scintiscan. It is wise to discontinue L-thyroxine in these patients because thyroid suppression leads only to trouble.

THYROID CARCINOMA
General Description

Pathologically, there are several forms of thyroid cancer, but clinically thyroid carcinoma has four varieties: (*a*) papillary or mixed papillary-follicular carcinoma (65–75% of all thyroid cancer); (*b*) follicular thyroid carcinoma (20–30%); (*c*) medullary thyroid carcinoma (5–10%); and (*d*) anaplastic carcinoma (which is rare, found in the elderly, responds poorly to any therapy, and is invariably fatal). Histology bears on the prognosis. Papillary and mixed papillary-follicular carcinoma behave similarly and have a benign course; follicular carcinoma is more aggressive. Age of the patient at the time of diagnosis is a major prognostic feature; in short the older the patient, the worse the prognosis. Young patients do well, and seldom is there death from papillary thyroid cancer below the age of 40. Papillary and mixed papillary-follicular cancers have a median age of onset of 35 years, whereas follicular thyroid carcinomas occur at a median age of 45 years. There is no difference in prognosis between men and women. An initial tumor larger than 4 cm, metastasis, and tumor invasion into muscle or trachea signal a poorer prognosis; however, metastasis of papillary or mixed papillary-follicular carcinoma to regional lymph glands does *not* adversely affect prognosis.

Medullary thyroid carcinoma (MTC) of the parafollicular or C cells is generally found at surgery for a solitary thyroid nodule (although it can be diagnosed before surgery by aspiration biopsy). MTC is a sporadic event in about 80% of cases, with the average patient age in the middle 50s. The remainder of cases are inherited as an autosomal dominant trait. MTC is associated with pheochromocytoma (50% of cases) and hyperparathyroidism (10–25% of the patients) in multiple endocrine neoplasia (MEN) type IIa. MTC with mucosal neuromatosis without hyperparathyroidism occurs in MEN type IIb or III. MTC associated with this latter syndrome (IIb) is very aggressive. Early detection of MTC in family members is possible and, with total thyroidectomy, represents the only way to cure this disease. Calcitonin, the biochemical marker of MTC, is elevated (>200 pg/mL) in patients with obvious disease. Before nodular disease, these patients have C cell hyperplasia. Provocative testing identifies this premalignant condition. Plasma calcitonin levels are drawn at 0 time and at 2, 3.5, 5, and 7 minutes after intravenous calcium gluconate (2 mg elemental calcium/kg over 1 minute) followed by a 10-second bolus of pentagastrin 0.5 μg/kg. A rise of >200 pg/mL is diagnostic of C cell hyperplasia or MTC. In the near future, family members of affected patients for MTC may be screened for the carrier state by assaying leukocytes for genetic markers of the disorder, thus avoiding the inconvenience, discomfort, and cost of repetitive pentagastrin stimulation.

Surgery is essential to prevent overt disease. Several factors affect the prognosis of MTC. (*a*) Type of MTC: MEN IIb-associated MTCs tend to be very aggressive (early metastases and infiltrating lesions), whereas non-MEN MTCs have a better prognosis. The biology of aggressiveness follows: MEN IIb > MEN IIa > sporadic MTC > non-MEN MTC. (*b*) Size of the primary mass correlates with prognosis (the larger the mass, the worse the outcome). (*c*) Level of plasma calcitonin: levels of calcitonin above 10,000 ng/mL are associated with high mortality. Lesser elevations of calcitonin are associated with higher survival rates. (*d*) Degree of calcitonin-immunoperoxidase staining of the tumor: high levels of reactivity (>75% staining) are associated with good prognosis. Low levels of staining predict poor outcome.

Management

Management of thyroid carcinoma spurs controversy among endocrinologists and surgeons. The rarity, protracted course, and low mortality of well-differentiated thyroid carcinoma have made randomized treatment regimens difficult to perform. It is generally agreed that the nodule should be removed and that thyroid suppressive therapy should be continued indefinitely. How much thyroid to remove (one lobe vs subtotal or total thyroidectomy) and the best method to provide follow-up are the unanswered variables. Individualized therapy should be based on the histology of the tumor, age of patient, and size and extent of the initial tumor. For follicular thyroid carcinoma (which frequently has vascular invasion), a more aggressive approach is advised. Total thyroidectomy or near total thyroidectomy followed by radioiodine ablation (29.9–100 mCi 131-iodine) 1–2 months after surgery while the patient is hypothyroid (i.e., on no replacement L-thyroxine) ablates any remaining functioning thyroid cells. Thyroid suppression with L-thyroxine is then instituted to ensure that serum TSH is low (0.1–0.3 μU/mL range). Functioning thyroid cells but not C cells produce thyroglobulin, which is found in the serum in small amounts. Once the thyroid is ablated, no serum thyroglobulin is detectable. The presence of any measurable serum thyroglobulin after total ablation suggests recurrence of the disease. Unfortunately, 10–20% of thyroid cancer patients have antibodies that interfere with thyroglobulin determinations, so one cannot reliably use this marker in these patients. Six months later (after L-thyroxine is discontinued for at least 1 month), a total body 131-iodine scan is performed as follows. The patient is given 1–5 mCi 131-iodine and then scintiscan 24 hours and 48 hours later. If the 6-month scan is negative, L-thyroxine suppression is reinstituted and the procedure repeated in 12–18 months. If negative, then scans are performed every 5 years unless there is evidence of local recurrence or the serum thyroglobulin levels rise. If functioning tissue is identified on any scan, then 131-iodine 100–200 mCi is given, L-thyroxine reinstituted, and the body scan repeated 6 months later. This course is repeated as long as the scan is positive. Patients who are to receive >30 mCi 131-iodine are hospitalized because of radiation safety standards. Patients are seen in yearly follow-up to assess the neck for recurrent nodules, check serum thyroglobulin, obtain chest X-ray (at least every 2–3 years), and to assure that serum TSH is suppressed with L-thyroxine.

The younger patient who has the 2-cm <u>papillary thyroid carcinoma</u> should be managed with a total or subtotal thyroidectomy and local lymph node resection with care to preserve parathyroid function followed by lifelong thyroid suppression. Local tumor recurrence occurs more frequently after unilateral lobectomy than with bilobar resection, probably related to the multicentric nature of papillary disease. Treating these patients with radioiodine ablation reduces the incidence of local nodal recurrence and is often done, but whether this improves prognosis is uncertain because these patients have excellent life expectancy. Any recurrent neck masses can be easily resected.

The only reason for less surgery (i.e., subtotal thyroidectomy) at the initial operation is to avoid possible damage to the parathyroid glands, which would render the patient chronically dependent on calcium and vitamin D (Chapter 12). Up to 20% incidence of permanent hypoparathyroidism has been reported with total thyroidectomy. This is not often a problem if the parathyroid glands are transplanted by an experienced surgeon.

Treatment of MTC is total thyroidectomy, ruling out pheochromocytoma (page 196) and hyperparathyroidism (page 162), and screening family members for the disease.

HYPERTHYROIDISM

Hyperthyroidism is the syndrome that develops after body tissues are exposed to increased concentrations of thyroxine (T4) and/or triiodothyronine (T3). Clinical manifestations of hyperthyroidism may affect every organ. The presentation varies with age; the classical symptoms and signs of hypermetabolism are seen in young and middle-aged patients but less so in the elderly. The degree of hyperthyroidism also varies with the severity of the levels of T4 and T3.

The symptoms of hyperthyroidism relate to <u>excessive sympathomimetic activity</u> and <u>increased catabolic activity</u>: nervousness (irritability and emotional lability); increased perspiration; heat intolerance; palpitations; weight loss; dyspnea; fatigue and weakness; increased appetite; hyperdefecation; menstrual dysfunction; and eye symptoms.

Signs of hyperthyroidism include goiter (thyroid enlargement), tremor, hyperkinesis, eye signs (exophthalmos, lid retraction, lid lag), tachycardia (resting rate >90; atrial fibrillation), smooth and velvety skin, moist and warm hands, onycholysis ("Plummer's nails"), and thyroid bruit. In the elderly these classical signs are often missing, and one sees cardiac problems (heart failure and tachydysrhythmias), weight loss, weakness, or anorexia. The striking absence of the adrenergic and hyperkinetic symptoms is sometimes called <u>apathetic hyperthyroidism</u>. When a patient with hyperthyroidism presents with fever, altered mental status, and acceleration of these signs and symptoms, the clinical diagnosis of thyroid storm is made ("Thyroid Storm," Chapter 2). Like thyroid diseases in general, hyperthyroidism is much more common in females than males.

The diagnosis of hyperthyroidism is very easy when the clinical disease is obvious. When the signs and symptoms are minimal, the laboratory is helpful. The serum T4(radioimmunoassay (RIA))/thyroid hormone binding index (T3U) or free T4 are usually elevated as is the serum T3(RIA). The T3(RIA) or free T3 is usually elevated to a greater extent than the T4(RIA) and is sometimes the only abnormal laboratory finding (i.e., T3 thyrotoxicosis). <u>Serum TSH levels are suppressed or nonmeasurable (<0.1 μU/mL).</u> Hyperthyroidism has generalized effects on various tissues producing numerous abnormal laboratory studies that revert to normal when the hyperthyroidism resolves. Such findings include hypercalcemia, abnormal liver function studies, and increased turnover and degradation of metabolites (e.g., an increase in urinary 17-hydroxycorticosteroid, making one suspect Cushing's syndrome). Subclinical hyperthyroidism is frequently detected by low levels of TSH on screening chemistry profiles. The radionuclide thyroid uptake or scan is not ordered to make a diagnosis of hyperthyroidism but is helpful in deciding etiology of the hyperthyroidism.

Hyperthyroidism has many causes. These are listed in order of decreasing frequency: (a) <u>Graves' disease</u>, (b) <u>thyroiditis</u>, (c) <u>toxic multinodular goiter</u>, (d) <u>toxic thyroid adenoma</u>, (e) <u>exogenous hyperthyroidism</u> (iatrogenic, factitious, iodine induced), (f) <u>excess TSH</u> (trophoblastic tumors, pituitary tumor), and (g) <u>ectopic T4 production</u> (struma ovarii and metastatic follicular thyroid carcinoma).

Graves' Disease

General Description

Graves' disease is by far the most common cause of hyperthyroidism, with a female-to-male ratio of 7:1 or 8:1. It is typically a disease of young women (ages 20–40 years) but may occur at any age. Graves' disease is distinguished clinically from other forms of hyperthyroidism by the presence of <u>diffuse thyroid enlargement</u>, <u>ophthalmopathy</u>, and occasionally pretibial myxedema, although all these signs may be absent. A thyroid bruit is heard only in this form of hyperthyroidism. Ophthalmopathy is present in 20–40% of patients with recent onset of Graves' disease and may develop before hyperthyroidism ("euthyroid Graves' disease"), at the onset of hyperthyroidism (the usual case), or years later after the patient is euthyroid.

Graves' disease is an immunologic disorder of uncertain cause. Mononuclear cells produce thyroid-stimulating immunoglobulins that bind to the TSH receptors on thyroid follicular cells, causing thyroidogenesis. When thyroid-stimulating immunoglobulin levels decrease for any cause (most often spontaneous), the hyperthyroidism goes into remission. What causes these activated mononuclear cells to turn on (and off in the case of remission) is unknown. Genetic factors are important since 50% of monozygotic twins are concordant for hyperthyroidism and 5% of first-degree relatives have a history of hyperthyroidism. Currently the treatment of Graves' disease is directed at the thyroid gland rather than at the basic process that initiates the clinical disease.

Treatment

The optimal therapy awaits a method that treats the cause of this disorder. The best one can now do is to control the hyperthyroidism with antithyroid drugs until the basic disease process undergoes spontaneous remission. Unfortunately spontaneous remission occurs in only 20–30% of patients in the United States. Therefore the clinician must decide on long-term antithyroid medication for 1–2 years or on some form of ablative thyroid therapy such as radioactive iodine or, much less frequently, subtotal thyroidectomy.

Antithyroid Drugs. The thionamides, propylthiouracil (PTU) and methimazole (Tapazole), block thyroid peroxidase and thus inhibit thyroid hormone biosynthesis. Both drugs have weak immunosuppressive effects, and PTU in high doses has an inhibitory effect on the conversion of T4 to T3. The half-life of PTU is 1–2 hours, whereas methimazole is 6–8 hours. Maximal effect is achieved with divided doses (every 6–8 hours), especially with PTU. There are no reliable markers to define the population that will undergo spontaneous remission while on thionamide therapy. Clinically there are two groups that respond well to long-term treatment—patients with a small thyroid gland and patients whose hyperthyroidism is of very recent onset. These patients are treated with PTU 100–300 mg tid or methimazole 10–30 mg every day until the serum T4 is normal (usually 6–8 weeks after initiation), and then the dose is reduced or L-thyroxine is added to maintain euthyroid status. Patients are maintained on this therapy for 1–2 years before the drug is discontinued, although remissions have been reported when the drug is discontinued earlier. One of the most difficult aspects of therapy is to maintain patient compliance in taking medications. This is especially difficult with PTU, which is only available as 50-mg tablets, taken three times a day. Single daily doses of methimazole 5–20 mg/day are a practical solution. Complications of thionamides are infrequent, with rash being the most common problem (about 5% of the patients). Agranulocytosis is the most dreaded complication (0.2% of patients). Routine blood counts are not helpful or predictive of this toxic effect. The best policy is to tell the patient to come immediately for a complete blood count if there is fever, sore throat, or diarrhea. Other toxic reactions such as fever, myalgia, lupus-like syndromes, and hepatitis occur but generally remit as soon as the drug is discontinued.

Children and adolescents are usually managed with long-term thionamide therapy. Although the case is made that radioactive therapy is safe for children with hyperthyroidism, this is not universally accepted. Thionamides are used in treating the hyperthyroidism during pregnancy with lower doses than if the patient was not pregnant. These antithyroid medications cross the placenta and if given in large doses inhibit the fetal thyroid gland. Doses of PTU up to 300 mg/day are generally safe. A mild degree of hyperthyroidism during pregnancy is usually well tolerated on thionamide treatment.

Short courses (1–3 months) of antithyroid drugs are used to reduce thyroid hormone levels and decrease the amount of hormone within the thyroid in preparation for ablative therapy.

Radioactive Iodine Therapy. 131-Iodine therapy is the treatment of choice for most adults with Graves' disease. Patients who have failed long-term thionamide are also treated with 131-iodine. It is safe, effective, convenient, and much less expensive than surgery; pregnancy is the only absolute contraindication. Most patients are treated as outpatients. Elderly or especially ill patients are treated with thionamides until euthyroid; then the thionamide is discontinued for 4–7 days and 131-iodine given. This reduces the amount of thyroid hormone released after radiation injury and avoids the cardiovascular effects that may occur with a sudden surge in the serum levels of thyroid hormones. Younger patients may be treated while they are still hyperthyroid and covered with β-adrenergic blockers (e.g., propranolol). The dose of 131-iodine is generally 5–15 mCi. The lower dose is associated with lower incidence of hypothyroidism but a higher incidence of unresolved hyperthyroidism. High doses of 131-iodine reverse these incidences. Within 6–12 weeks after 131-iodine the patient is generally euthyroid, and treatment with propranolol is discontinued. If the patient is still hyperthyroid 6 months after 131-iodine, a second treatment is necessary. The incidence of hypothyroidism that develops depends on treatment dose and ranges from 20 to 70%. Surveillance for hypothyroidism must be lifelong. Practically, it is easier to manage the patient if there is good ablation leading to early hypothyroidism. This complication is acceptable since thyroid hormone replacement is easily managed with L-thyroxine 0.075–0.15 mg/day at a cost of ≤20¢/day. Good follow-up is necessary to treat hypothyroidism early or to detect the recurrence of hyperthyroidism.

Surgery. Subtotal thyroidectomy is infrequently used in the treatment of hyperthyroidism. Children who fail with thionamides or patients who refuse radioactive medications for personal reasons and the occasionally pregnant patient with hyperthyroidism who cannot be managed with acceptable doses of thionamides are treated with surgery. Before operation, the patient is made euthyroid with thionamides and potassium iodide drops. Pregnant patients are not given the customary iodine preparation to reduce thyroid vascularity because large fetal goiters may result.

β-Adrenergic Antagonists. The introduction of β-adrenergic antagonists has had a major influence of the management of hyperthyroidism. Propranolol is the most commonly used blocker. Propranolol alleviates but does not totally resolve many symptoms of hyperthyroidism such as tachycardia, sweating, tremor, heat intolerance, and anxiety. The usual dose is 20–40 mg qid. As mentioned above, propranolol is used as an adjunct to treatment with 131-iodine until the therapeutic effect of 131-iodine is achieved. It is also used in conjunction with potassium iodine and thionamides in preparing patients with hyperthyroidism for surgery. Propranolol is not prescribed if there is asthma. Propranolol is especially useful in the treatment of thyroid storm ("Thyroid Storm," Chapter 2).

Iodine. Inorganic iodine inhibits thyroid hormone synthesis and release. Traditional doses of 5–10 drops of saturated solution of potassium iodine three times a day in water or juice reduce serum T4 and T3 by 50% within 7–14 days. Then, T4 and T3 levels return to previous levels in most patients. This escape phenomenon does not occur in a previously damaged thyroid (e.g., radiation injury) and thus is useful following 131-iodine therapy. Iodine is also used before surgery in hyperthyroid subjects who are not pregnant.

Thyroiditis

Two forms of thyroiditis may cause hyperthyroidism: subacute (de Quervain's, granulomatous, or giant-cell) thyroiditis and painless thyroiditis. <u>Subacute thyroiditis</u> is a painful condition that often follows some respiratory illness. Thyroid follicles are disrupted, and stored hormone is released, causing hyperthyroid symptoms in 50% of the patients, although levels of T4 are elevated in an even higher percentage. The radionuclide thyroid uptake is characteristically very low (1–2% at 24 hours) early in this disorder. The hyperthyroidism is self-limited, lasting for only a few weeks. <u>Thionamides are not indicated and do not work.</u> Propranolol 20–40 mg qid is used for the hyperthyroid patient. Aspirin 650 mg qid is prescribed for treatment of the pain and is continued for several weeks after the pain resolves in an attempt to prevent recurrence of pain. If the pain is protracted or there is significant fever unresponsive to aspirin, prednisone 20–40 mg/day is used for 1–2 weeks, after which the dose is gradually tapered for 2–4 weeks to avoid flare up. <u>Painless thyroiditis</u> appears to be an increasing cause of hyperthyroidism. The gland is nontender and only slightly enlarged. The radionuclide thyroid uptake is usually low but may be normal or increased if the process is healing or resolving. Etiology is uncertain. Treatment is the same as subacute thyroiditis except that salicylates and/or steroids are omitted.

Toxic Multinodular Goiter

Hyperthyroidism may develop as a late feature of multinodular goiter. Areas within the goiter become autonomous, i.e., not responsive to TSH. If sufficient amount of tissue functions excessively, hyperthyroidism develops. The mechanism responsible for the autonomy is unknown. This is a disease of elderly patients (typically females older than 60 years). Large goiters may present with occasional retrosternal extension and tracheal compression. Many times the hyperthyroidism is mild, and symptoms may be masked (apathetic hyperthyroidism). Cardiac failure and atrial fibrillation may be present. The radionuclide scan shows patchy areas of increased activity. At times these patients become hyperthyroid after ingestion of organic iodine (often with T3 thyrotoxicosis). Others become toxic during thyroid suppressive therapy instituted to reduce the size of the goiter. In the latter two instances removing the offending agent is the first therapeutic move.

Toxic multinodular goiter is treated with ablative 131-iodine therapy or surgery. Patients are first given antithyroid medication to achieve euthyroidism. Thionamides are not prescribed for long-term therapy since spontaneous remissions rarely, if ever, occur. Large doses of 131-iodine (30 mCi) are necessary to ablate the thyroid, and multiple doses are often necessary to control the hyperthyroidism. Surgery is preferred for large goiters producing obstructive symptoms.

Toxic Adenoma

Toxic thyroid adenoma is a solitary benign lesion (follicular adenoma) that functions autonomously. The natural history is that of slow progressive growth except for an occasional tumor necrosis that leads to a decrease in nodule size. Whether the patient becomes hyperthyroid depends on the size of the nodule. The nodule usually has to be >4 cm for hyperthyroidism to be evident. Smaller nodules may be hyperfunctioning on scan and produce enough thyroid hormone to suppress TSH and therefore reduce the uptake of radionuclide in surrounding normal thyroid tissue. T3 hyperthyroidism occurs in up to 50% of these patients.

Treatment is with <u>surgery</u> or <u>radioactive iodine</u>. For patients younger than 40 years, surgery is recommended for those who have overt hyperthyroidism and prophylactically for those with large nodules. Hyperthyroid patients are prepared for surgery either with antithyroid drugs or with the combination of propranolol and inorganic iodine. Many older patients receive 131-iodine therapy. Large doses of 131-iodine (20–30 mCi) are necessary to ablate the adenoma. Hypothyroidism is less common after 131-iodine therapy for toxic thyroid adenoma and toxic multinodular goiter, whereas it is the rule after treatment for Graves' disease. Smaller autonomous nodules in euthyroid patients need not be treated, but the patients must be followed carefully and thyroid function measured at yearly intervals.

Exogenous Hyperthyroidism

The following three causes of hyperthyroidism relate to ingestion of excessive amounts of thyroid hormone or iodine preparations.

Iatrogenic Hyperthyroidism

This condition develops in patients receiving larger than replacement doses of thyroid hormones. This is common with doses of L-thyroxine in excess of 0.2 mg and is even more common when T3 or a combination T4 and T3 is used. Assessment of the thyroid status by measuring serum T4 may be misleading in patients treated with T3 or combined T3-T4 preparations. Occasional patients with multinodular goiter on seemingly appropriate suppressive doses of L-thyroxine (e.g., 0.125 mg/day) may have high T4 levels. This is the time to determine whether there is autonomous function within the adenomatous nodules (contributing to the hyperthyroxinemia) or whether the dose of L-thyroxine itself is too much. A radionuclide uptake and scan should be performed. If the uptake is >5% or if functioning nodule(s) is found, L-thyroxine is discontinued. If the uptake is <5% and no hyperfunctioning areas are identified, then the dose of L-thyroxine is reduced.

Factitious Hyperthyroidism

Some patients with personality disorders (often paramedical personnel) may induce hyperthyroidism by the intentional self-administration of thyroid hormones. In these cases, the thyroid gland is not enlarged, nor are there any signs of ophthalmopathy or pretibial myxedema. The serum T4(RIA), T3(RIA), or both are elevated depending on which thyroid hormone preparation is ingested. Serum TSH is suppressed, and the radionuclide thyroid uptake is low. Furthermore, the serum thyroglobulin is low where it is increased in patients with thyroiditis who also have a low thyroid uptake. Psychiatric referral may be necessary for these patients.

Iodine-Induced Hyperthyroidism (Jod-Basedow Phenomenon)

In areas of endemic goiter caused by iodine deficiency, dietary iodine supplementation decreases the size of the thyroid. Nevertheless, this treatment induces hyperthyroidism in a subset of patients who have a preexisting thyroid abnormality. Iodine-induced hyperthyroidism also occurs in nonendemic regions in patients who have multinodular goiter or thyroid adenoma. These patients become hyperthyroid several weeks after ingestion of large doses of inorganic iodine (e.g., amiodarone) or radiographic contrast agents. Because the pool of iodine is expanded, the radionuclide thyroid uptake may be low. Symptomatic treatment with propranolol and withdrawal of any iodine-containing medication are indicated.

Excessive TSH

TSH producing tumors are a very rare cause of hyperthyroidism. About 100 cases of a pituitary tumor producing TSH have been re-

Table 11.1
Features of Common Types of Hyperthyroidism

	Graves' Disease	Toxic Nodular Goiter	Iodine-Induced Hyperthyroidism
Age of onset (yr)	10–40	50–70	40–70
Onset of symptoms	Insidious	Insidious	Acute
Family history	Frequent	Infrequent	Rare
Goiter (%)	97	100	75
Character of goiter	Diffuse	Nodular	Variable (often multinodular)
Exophthalmos	Frequent	Rare	Rare
Thyroid uptake	Elevated	Usually elevated	Decreased
Thyroid scintiscan	Diffuse	Areas of increased uptake	Cannot visualize
Associated autoimmune disease	Frequent	Rare	Rare
Thyroid antibodies	Often present	Absent	Infrequent
Spontaneous remission	May occur	Rare	Usually resolves after iodine withdrawal

ported; most since the TSH assay has been a standard test in evaluating hyperthyroid patients. Trophoblastic tumors such as choriocarcinoma, hydatidiform moles, or embryonal carcinoma of the testes produce high levels of chorionic gonadotropin that weakly cross react with the TSH receptor of the thyroid follicular cell. In these cases, overt hyperthyroidism is rare.

Ectopic Thyroid Hormone Production

On very rare occasions, hyperthyroidism may be caused by production of thyroid hormone from the ovary (struma ovarii) or from metastatic follicular thyroid carcinoma.

Table 11.1 summarizes the features of common types of hyperthyroidism.

HYPOTHYROIDISM

Hypothyroidism develops when there is an inadequate effect of thyroid hormone on body tissues. Greater than 99.9% of the time, hypothyroidism is caused by deficient production of thyroid hormones by the thyroid gland, leading to low serum levels of T4. Very rarely hypothyroidism is due to failure of tissues to respond to normal or raised levels of thyroid hormones (i.e., peripheral resistance). In hypothyroidism the tissues are infiltrated by hydrophilic mucopolysaccharides. This leads to the nonpitting edema (most marked in the skin of the eyelids and hands) termed myxedema.

The clinical spectrum of hypothyroidism ranges from subtle and subclinical disease to gross and obvious changes that have developed over years. Classical symptoms of hypothyroidism include the following: marked cold intolerance (prefers warm room, extra clothes, sleeps with blanket during warm months); weakness (increased tiredness, slowing down); muscle cramps, aching, and stiffness; hoarseness, decreased hearing, and paresthesia (a result of myxedematous changes in the vocal cords, middle ear and eighth cranial nerve, and carpal tunnel syndrome, respectively); mild weight gain despite normal appetite; constipation and ileus; dry skin and decreased perspiration; and somnolence. Frequent signs include skin that is rough, scaly, dry, cool to the touch, and pallid or yellow tinted (the result of anemia or hypercarotenemia owing to impaired conversion of carotene to vitamin A); nonpitting edema of the eyelids, hands, and feet; slow movements and slowness of thought (a dementia that responds to T4 replacement); slow relaxation time of deep tendon reflexes; and cardiovascular signs (bradycardia, cardiac failure, pericardial effusion, and hypertension). Severe hypothyroidism can lead to coma and respiratory compromise ("Myxedema Coma," Chapter 2). Congenital hypothyroidism is associated with mental retardation and characteristic facies. Juvenile hypothyroidism is characterized by epiphyseal dysgenesis and short stature. Goiter may be present depending on etiology of the hypothyroidism.

Etiology

Hypothyroidism has many causes, but most involve thyroid (primary) hypofunction either with insufficient amount of functional tissue (e.g., primary atrophy, chronic thyroiditis, prior 131-iodine treatment or surgery, or thyroid agenesis) or some form of defective biosynthesis of thyroid hormone (e.g., iodine deficiency, congenital defects of trapping or organification of iodine, excessive antithyroid medications, or iodine excess). Secondary hypothyroidism related to pituitary disease (e.g., pituitary tumor) is usually but not always obvious because other signs of hypopituitarism are often present. If the serum T4 and T3U are low and the TSH is low as well, one should examine the hypothalamic-pituitary axis. Clinically, primary hypothyroidism can be classified by whether a <u>goiter is present and by whether the hypothyroidism follows some ablative procedure</u>.

Nongoitrous Hypothyroidism

<u>Spontaneous primary thyroid atrophy</u> is a common cause of hypothyroidism. <u>No goiter is present.</u> It is found more often in females than males (6:1) and increases in frequency with age. There is loss of thyroid tissue as a result of autoimmune destruction leading to fibrosis and atrophy of the thyroid. Primary atrophy represents one end of the spectrum of autoimmune thyroid disease; at the other is chronic autoimmune (Hashimoto's) thyroiditis in which there is marked proliferation of lymphocytes and acinar formation leading to goiter. In most cases thyroid failure has been present for months or years before diagnosis. There may be associated failure of other endocrine organs, including pernicious anemia, diabetes mellitus, hypogonadism, hypoparathyroidism, and Addison's disease.

Goitrous Hypothyroidism

<u>Chronic autoimmune thyroiditis (Hashimoto's thyroiditis)</u> is characterized by a diffuse enlargement of the thyroid gland and high titers of thyroid autoantibodies. This condition is the most common cause of goitrous hypothyroidism in iodine-replete parts of the world. Titers of autoantibodies are much higher than in primary thyroid atrophy. Histologically the thyroid has large amounts of lymphocyte infiltration with areas of marked follicular hypertrophy and/or numerous oxyphilic cells (Askanazy or Hürthle cells). Failure of other endocrine organs may be associated with Hashimoto's thyroiditis. For example, the combination of chronic lymphocytic thyroiditis and idiopathic adrenal insufficiency is known as Schmidt's syndrome.

Postablative Hypothyroidism

This condition may follow surgery or radioactive iodine therapy and represents a frequent cause of hypothyroidism. In fact, post 131-iodine induced hypothyroidism is the most common cause of hypothyroidism in my clinic.

Other Types of Hypothyroidism

<u>Drug-induced hypothyroidism</u> may be secondary to lithium carbonate, iodine, or antithyroid drugs. Lithium inhibits the release of thy-

roid hormone and is one of the common causes of goiter but rarely causes hypothyroidism. Iodine may cause goiter in susceptible subjects (i.e., those with some underlying thyroid abnormality) and lead to hypothyroidism. Typically this is seen in patients with chronic respiratory disease taking expectorants containing potassium iodide.

Hypothyroidism caused by iodine deficiency is a common problem in areas of endemic goiter in certain parts of the world. It is almost never seen in the United States.

Inherited disorders of dyshormonogenesis are rare and are typically inherited as an autosomal recessive trait. The most common defect is associated with progressive hearing loss leading to deafness and goiter owing to an inability to organify iodine (Pendred's syndrome).

Laboratory Studies

Hypothyroidism is confirmed by finding a low serum T4 and T3U or low serum free T4. In all forms of primary hypothyroidism the serum TSH is elevated and should always be measured since a low value implies pituitary disease. Antibodies to thyroid microsomes and thyroglobulin are usually present in autoimmune thyroid disease (primary atrophy and Hashimoto's thyroiditis). Anemia of some form (microcytic, from menstrual loss in premenopausal females; normochromic normocytic, from decreased erythropoietin production; macrocytic, from associated pernicious anemia) is often present. Clearance of the enzymes, creatine kinase and aspartate aminotransferase, is reduced and may be markedly elevated in the serum. Serum cholesterol and triglycerides are often raised. The sella turcica may be enlarged in long-term hypothyroidism, particularly in children and adolescents. The ECG may demonstrate low voltage if pericardial effusion is present. Serum T3(RIA) or free T3 levels are not helpful because over half of the patients with hypothyroidism have levels within the normal range.

Treatment of Hypothyroidism

Therapy for primary hypothyroidism is simple. L-thyroxine routinely prescribed in a dose of 0.75 μg/lb body weight/day; the average replacement dose is 125 μg (0.075–0.15 mg)/day. The half-life of T4 is 6–8 days, which allows for stable and constant serum levels of T4. The advantages of synthetic L-thyroxine include the following: assured potency; single daily dose; inexpensive (≤20¢/day); constant levels of serum T4; and the ability to assess adequacy of replacement by measuring serum TSH. Absorption of L-thyroxine is somewhat variable among individuals. Most patients normalize their TSH with 0.125 mg L-thyroxine/day and nearly all with 0.15 mg/day. Since 80% of body T3 is derived by conversion of T4, serum T3(RIA) levels are normal in the patient taking replacement L-thyroxine.

The regimen for each patient must be individualized. For the young, mildly hypothyroid patient one may start with the full replacement dose (e.g., L-thyroxine 0.125 mg/day), remembering that it will take 4–6 weeks for the full effects of T4 to be realized. For the severely hypothyroid patient, gradual replacement is indicated to avoid cardiovascular problems. L-thyroxine 0.025 mg/day is prescribed for 2 weeks and then increased by 0.025 mg/day every 2 weeks until a maintenance dose is reached. The goal is to have serum TSH levels in the normal range. Before changing the dose of L-thyroxine, the patient should be on the same dose for at least 4–6 weeks. Checking the TSH more frequently is not informative and wastes money.

T3 is not routinely used for several reasons: peaks of T3 after gut absorption are much higher than normal serum T3(RIA); T3 must be taken three times a day; T3 is considerably more expensive than L-thyroxine; and serum TSH cannot reliably be used to assess replacement therapy.

A problem with all medications that must be taken chronically is patient compliance. Education regarding the importance of renewing prescriptions and annual follow-up to assess long-term therapy cannot be overemphasized. Remember that certain medications affect absorption of T4 (e.g., bile resin binders, iron, sucralfate). Elderly hypothyroid patients may forget to take their medications, so it is important that someone be responsible for them to avoid this problem. Using a "pill box" in which daily medications are placed helps.

MISCELLANEOUS THYROID STATES
Withdrawal of Thyroid Medication

There are large numbers of patients who have had thyroid medication prescribed for vague symptoms (e.g., weakness, fatigue, menstrual dysfunction) without any laboratory documentation of hypothyroidism. The best way to find out whether the patient needs to continue thyroid medications is to discontinue the preparation; 6 weeks later measure serum T4/T3U, FT4, and TSH. If the patient is symptomatic *and* the laboratory values confirm hypothyroidism, then reinstitute thyroid using L-thyroxine as discussed above. If the patient has no symptoms and the TSH is slightly elevated, wait several more weeks until symptoms develop and TSH remains elevated before starting L-thyroxine. If the laboratory values are normal 6 weeks after discontinuing thyroid preparation, no further medication is prescribed. Follow-up 3–6 months later should confirm that no replacement is necessary.

Simple Nontoxic Goiter

Simple goiter is found often in young women who present with enlargement of the anterior neck. The thyroid may be just palpable or moderately enlarged. The gland is usually soft, nontender, and diffusely enlarged. No nodules are palpable. The patient is asymptomatic and is chemically euthyroid. Thyroid autoantibodies are absent or present in low titer. The etiology is rarely discernible. The patient may be merely followed to see if the thyroid will continue to enlarge or may be begun on thyroid suppression if the gland is already modestly enlarged. Thyroid suppression will usually decrease the size of the thyroid, and therapy is continued indefinitely. Inform the patient that discontinuation of thyroid medications may be followed by recurrence of the goiter.

Pseudogoiter

Pseudogoiter exists when any fullness in the neck leads the physician to make a diagnosis of goiter when, in fact, an enlarged thyroid is not present. In most cases, pseudogoiter represents prominent adipose tissue (fat pad goiter). When a normal sized thyroid gland is located more superiorly in the neck, it becomes more prominent, leading to a diagnosis of pseudogoiter secondary to a high lying thyroid. A high lying thyroid may be diagnosed by an experienced clinician who palpates the thyroid to be normal in size. On radionuclide scan the anterior view demonstrates the midpoint of the isthmus lying more than 60% of the way from the suprasternal notch to the superior notch of the thyroid cartilage. Rarely, a delphian node (located between the hyoid bone and thyroid cartilage), dermoid cyst, parathyroid cyst, laryngeal lesion, or lipoma might present as pseudogoiter.

Euthyroid Sick

Thyroid tests are often ordered to screen for thyroid disease in patients who have weakness, anxiety, tachycardia, and weight loss. Most of these patients do *not* have primary thyroid disease. Euthyroid sick is a term designated for those patients with nonthyroid illnesses who have abnormal thyroid tests and can be classified into the following categories: (*a*) low T3 syndrome; (*b*) low T3 and low T4 syndrome; (*c*) high T4 syndrome; and (*d*) a mixed form in which a combination of abnormalities may be found.

Low T3 syndrome is the most common of the euthyroid sick abnormalities but is usually not identified because most screening studies do not measure serum T3(RIA) or free T3. The serum T3/free T3 is low, and the serum T4(RIA) is normal. The patient is clinically euthyroid. Serum T3(RIA) may be low in many circumstances: systemic illnesses (e.g., liver disease, acute febrile illnesses, renal failure, neoplastic disorders, burns, and congestive heart failure); starvation; major surgery; and after taking some drugs (dexamethasone, cholecystographic dyes, amiodarone, high doses of propranolol, and thionamides). The common factor in all these conditions is reduced extrathyroidal conversion of T4 to T3. The conversion of reverse T3 to T2 is impaired, leading to increased levels of serum reverse T3. TSH is normal, and free T4 measured by dialysis techniques is normal or high. The low T3 resolves when the underlying illness clears.

The low T3 and low T4 syndrome is usually identified because a low serum T4 is found on screening for thyroid disease in sick patients. The free thyroid index is often low as well. These patients are severely ill, and the clinical assessment to totally exclude hypothyroidism is difficult. However, careful history and physical examination will *not* reveal the typical features of hypothyroidism (page 153). Free T4 levels are minimally low, normal, or high. Depending when blood is taken in the patient's illness, the serum TSH may be low, normal, or elevated (usually <20 µU/mL). Early in sickness, the TSH is normal to low; as the illness worsens, the TSH is often low, and as recovery ensues, the TSH is often above normal. Patients who have a low T3 and low T4 generally do not do well. When the T4(RIA) is <3 µg/dL, mortality approaches 84%, which underscores the severity of the nonthyroid illness found in this set of patients. There is no evidence that treatment with L-thyroxine helps these patients. In fact, most experts believe the low T4 and low T3 levels are an adaptive mechanism to spare protein catabolism under these circumstances. Being patient and checking thyroid function weeks after the illness resolves are the best treatment for euthyroid sick patients.

The major cause of elevated T4 (high T4 syndrome) in euthyroid sick patients is increased concentrations of thyroid-binding globulin produced in certain liver diseases (e.g., acute viral hepatitis, chronic active hepatitis, and primary biliary cirrhosis) and acute intermittent porphyria. Hyperthyroxinemia can be found in patients who have recently ingested radiographic contrast agents (ipodate (Oragrafin) or iopanoic acid (Telepaque)). These agents compete with 5'deiodinase and impair T4 to T3 conversion, which leads to elevated serum T4 levels. T4 returns to normal within 6–8 weeks. High doses of propranolol occasionally cause an elevated T4 presumably by inhibiting the conversion of T4 to T3.

Another cause of hyperthyroxinemia in which there is no evidence of clinical hyperthyroidism is familial dysalbuminemic hyperthyroxinemia, a disorder in which albumin binds T4 abnormally, leading to raised levels of T4(RIA) and normal T3U. Serum TSH and thyroid-releasing hormone study are normal in each of these conditions of elevated T4.

Suggested Readings

Burch W: A method of fine-needle aspiration thyroid biopsy. *Ann Intern Med* 98:1023, 1983.

Campbell NRC, Hasinorff BB, Stalts H, et al: Ferrous sulfate reduces thyroxine efficiency in patients with hypothyroidism. *Ann Intern Med* 117:1010, 1992.

Chopra IJ: Thyroid function in nonthyroidal illnesses. *Ann Intern Med* 98:946, 1983.

DeGroot LJ, Larsen PR, Refetoff S, Stanbury JB. Graves' disease and the manifestations of thyrotoxicosis. *The Thyroid and Its Diseases,* ed 5. New York, Wiley, 1984, pp 341–398.

Fradkin JE, Wolff J: Iodide-induced thyrotoxicosis. *Medicine* 62:1, 1983.

Gharib H, Goellner JR: Fine-needle aspiration of the thyroid: an appraisal. *Ann Intern Med* 118:282, 1993.

Hay ID: Papillary thyroid carcinoma: prediction of outcome in 1,500 consecutive patients treated at the Mayo Clinic during 1945–1985. *Endocrinol Metab Clin North Am* 19:545, 1990.

Ingbar SH. The thyroid gland. In Wilson JD, Foster DW (eds): *Textbook of Endocrinology,* ed 7. Philadelphia, Saunders, 1985, pp 682–815.

Larsen PR, Refetoff S, Stanbury JB. Thyroid neoplasia. *The Thyroid and Its Diseases,* ed 5. New York, Wiley, 1984, pp 756–831.

Mazzaferri EL: Papillary thyroid carcinoma: factors influencing prognosis and current therapy. *Semin Oncol* 14:315, 1987.

Mazzaferri EL: Management of a solitary thyroid nodule. *N Engl J Med* 328:553, 1993.

Peake RL: Recurrent apathetic hyperthyroidism. *Arch Intern Med* 141:258, 1981.

Ruiz M, Rajatanavin R, Young RA, et al: Familial dysalbuminemic hyperthyroxinemia: a syndrome that can be confused with thyrotoxicosis. *N Engl J Med* 306:635, 1982.

Saad MF, Ordonez NG, Rashid RK, et al: Medullary carcinoma of thyroid. *Medicine* 63:319, 1984.

Utiger RD: The thyroid: physiology, hyperthyroidism, hypothyroidism, and the painful thyroid. In Felig P, Baxter JD, Broadus AE, Frohman LA (eds): *Endocrinology and Metabolism,* ed 2. New York, McGraw-Hill, 1986, pp 389–472.

Wells SA Jr, Dilley WD, Farndon JA, et al: Early diagnosis and treatment of medullary thyroid carcinoma. *Arch Intern Med* 145:1248, 1984.

Chapter 12

Calcium Disorders

HYPERCALCEMIA

Normal serum calcium ranges from 8.5 to 10.2 mg/dL in most laboratories. Care should be taken to interpret serum calcium in view of the protein concentration, as discussed on page 24. Most patients with hypercalcemia are asymptomatic and are identified by the serendipitous finding of an elevated serum calcium on biochemical screening. Others present with symptoms and signs that can be directly attributed to an underlying disease (e.g., bone pain related to osseous metastasis or renal stones caused by hyperparathyroidism).

Symptoms of hypercalcemia relate to the degree and duration of the hypercalcemia. Patients with serum calcium levels below 11.0 mg/dL are rarely symptomatic regarding calcium itself, although they may be very symptomatic related to any underlying disease (e.g., malignancy). Levels of serum calcium between 11.0 and 14.0 mg/dL may be associated with symptoms. Hypercalcemia above 14.0 mg/dL is invariably associated with symptoms, and the risk of developing severe organ damage is significant at these levels. Symptoms of hypercalcemia are not specific. General symptoms of weakness, fatigue, and impaired mental concentration are frequent. Polyuria is an early manifestation; hypercalcemia impairs the ability of the renal tubules to respond to vasopressin (antidiuretic hormone), so urine cannot be maximally concentrated. Neurological symptoms of poor recent memory, depression, muscle weakness, and lethargy can progress to stupor and coma. Gastrointestinal complaints include anorexia, nausea, vomiting, and constipation.

Signs of hypercalcemia are uncommon or nonspecific. Band keratopathy, a manifestation of metastatic calcification, is probably the most specific sign of chronic hypercalcemia. Band keratopathy occurs in the medial and lateral margins of the cornea adjacent to the scleral

limbus, whereas deposition of arcus senilis begins superiorly and infe-
riorly and extends around the margins of the cornea giving the arcus
circularis (annulus senilis). Arcus circularis is separated from the limbus by a clear space within the cornea. This space is often obliterated
and filled with whitish deposits in band keratopathy. The predominant cardiovascular sign of hypercalcemia is hypertension. Shortened
QT interval on the ECG and increased sensitivity to digitalis are also
seen. Renal signs relate to the inability to concentrate urine, renal
stones, and renal insufficiency. Pancreatitis and peptic ulcer disease
are associated with hypercalcemia, as are gout and pseudogout.
Dehydration leading to hypercalcemic crisis (page 37) may be the only
sign of severe hypercalcemia.

Hypercalcemia has multiple etiologies. Greater than 90% of patients have either primary hyperparathyroidism or malignancy as the
cause of hypercalcemia. Other causes are listed in Table 12.1.

Hyperparathyroidism

The prevalence of hyperparathyroidism is about 1 in 1000. This disease affects females more often than males in a ratio of about 2:1 to
3:1. Most patients are older than 50 years. Hyperparathyroidism is
caused by a parathyroid adenoma in about 85% of the cases, by hyperplasia of the parathyroid glands (15%), or rarely by parathyroid
carcinoma. Before the introduction of screening serum profiles, clinical clues to hyperparathyroidism related to renal stones (64% of
cases), bone disease such as osteitis fibrosa cystica (about 20% of
cases), peptic ulcer disease (12% of cases), or hypertension (6% of
cases). Asymptomatic patients comprised about 7% of these cases.
These complications of parathyroid hormone (PTH) excess are still
seen, but the frequency of each has changed because patients are
identified earlier before such manifestations are evident. It is known
that primary hyperparathyroidism is a chronic disease and that patients can have asymptomatic hypercalcemia for years.

The diagnosis of hyperparathyroidism depends on demonstrating
persistent hypercalcemia in the absence of other causes of hypercalcemia. A history of hypercalcemia for more than a year in the absence
of weight loss and other systemic symptoms excludes the other major
cause of hypercalcemia, neoplastic disease. Records of previous laboratory studies are well worth the trouble of obtaining to see if prior hypercalcemia can be documented. An elevated serum PTH (page 24)
confirms the diagnosis. In 85–90% of patients with proven primary

Table 12.1
Causes of Hypercalcemia

Primary hyperparathyroidism
   Sporadic (90–95% of the cases of hyperparathyroidism)
   Familial syndromes (MEN I and MEN IIa)
      MEN I (tumors of pituitary, pancreas, and parathyroid)
      MEN IIa (medullary thyroid carcinoma, hyperparathyroidism,
        pheochromocytoma)
Neoplastic diseases
   Local osteolysis (breast and lung carcinoma metastatic to bone and
      myeloma)
   Humoral hypercalcemia of malignancy
Endocrine disorders
   Hyperthyroidism
   Adrenal insufficiency
   Familial hypocalciuric hypercalcemia
Medications
   Thiazide diuretics
   Vitamin D and rarely vitamin A intoxication
   Milk-alkali syndrome
   Phosphodiesterase inhibitors (e.g., theophylline)
   Lithium
Granulomatous diseases
   Sarcoidosis
   Beryllosis, tuberculosis, coccidiodomycosis
Miscellaneous
   Immobilization (associated with high bone turnover rates such as in
      Paget's disease)
   Recovery phase of acute renal failure (rare)
   Idiopathic hypercalcemia of infancy (rare)
   Dehydration

hyperparathyroidism, the absolute level of PTH is above normal; in the remainder the PTH is inappropriately elevated for the degree of hypercalcemia. Recognize that serum PTH levels in some PTH assays (usually not the intact PTH) rise in renal insufficiency. Other biochemical studies that are helpful but not diagnostic include hypophosphatemia (<3.0 mg/dL), serum chloride >106 mEq/L, serum chloride-to-serum phosphorus ratio of >33, elevated serum alkaline phosphatase, or a calcium-phosphate renal stone. Phosphate excretion and nephrogenous cyclic AMP are increased, but these studies are not necessary. Radiographic findings are rare in the asymptomatic patient, but subperiosteal resorption of the phalanges and metacarpals is virtually pathognomonic of hyperparathyroidism.

The only effective therapy for hyperparathyroidism is surgical removal of the parathyroid adenoma/hyperplasia. Severe hypercalcemia (serum calcium >12.0 mg/dL), renal disease, renal stones, and bone pain are indications for neck exploration. Likewise, patients with multiple endocrine neoplasia I and IIa who have hypercalcemia should have parathyroidectomy. Although the natural history for asymptomatic patients with lesser degrees of hypercalcemia (<12 mg/dL) is unknown, at least 25% of these patients develop some complication attributable to hyperparathyroidism (e.g., decreased creatinine clearance, renal stone, nephrocalcinosis, hypertension, etc.) within 5 years of follow-up. Unfortunately there is no marker to define which patients will develop these complications related to hypercalcemia. Controversy abounds regarding when to recommend surgery for the "asymptomatic" patient with minimal hypercalcemia. Younger patients, patients with nonspecific symptoms (e.g., aches, mental changes), patients with hypercalciuria (24-hour urine calcium >4 mg/kg), and women with decreased bone mineral content (forearm bone density decreases before lumbar spine) should be offered surgery. The critical factor in management of hyperparathyroidism is the availability of an experienced parathyroid surgeon. The surgeon must identify each parathyroid gland. Removal of the single enlarged gland (adenoma) or removal of 3.5 hyperplastic glands effectively manages the hypercalcemia. About 95% of patients are discharged cured on the 2nd or 3rd postoperative day. Age itself is not a contraindication to surgery. Hypocalcemia can be a problem after surgery, particularly in the patient who has preoperative bone disease and elevated serum alkaline phosphatase. Such patients generally need intravenous calcium in the immediate postoperative period and oral calcium (and possibly short-acting calcitriol 0.5–1.0 μg bid) for several weeks after the operation until the "hungry bones" have reached a state of equilibrium after escaping the resorptive effects of chronic hyperparathyroidism. By then the serum alkaline phosphatase and serum phosphorus will have returned to normal, and calcium supplementation can be discontinued. Persistent hypercalcemia usually means an adenoma in ectopic location (intrathyroidal, intrathymic, superior mediastinum, esophageal groove). The best procedure to localize persistent disease is sestamibi radionuclide scan. Recurrence of hyperparathyroidism is most likely in the patients with parathyroid hyperplasia (often the familial syndromes associated with hypercalcemia). Rarely (<1%) the hyperparathyroidism is due to parathyroid carcinoma; the only preoperative clues are a palpable neck mass and that the hypercalcemia may be more severe and PTH levels higher than in benign disease.

There is no satisfactory medical therapy for primary hyperparathyroidism. However, medical therapy is used in two well-defined areas. Life-threatening hypercalcemia is managed medically with hydration and agents that acutely lower serum calcium (pages 37–39). Patients who are unacceptable surgical risks are medically treated. Many of these patients have no symptoms directly related to hypercalcemia as long as adequate hydration is assured. Any illness such as viral gastroenteritis can lead to dehydration and hypercalcemic crisis, and the patient must be warned to get medical attention. Oral phosphates given initially in small doses to avoid diarrhea and increased to 1–2 g qid are reasonable agents to use in an attempt to lower the serum calcium. Careful monitoring of renal function, serum potassium, and serum phosphorus (maintained below 5 mg/dL to minimize ectopic calcification) is necessary. Estrogen (Premarin 0.625–1.25 mg/day) may be used because estrogen is known to inhibit PTH-induced bone resorption. Despite these measures there is no ideal medical therapy for these hypercalcemic patients who often have underlying illnesses such as hypertension or congestive heart failure that complicate therapy with salt loading and digitalis.

Neoplastic Diseases

For the hospitalized patient, hypercalcemia is most often due to malignancy. Malignancy may affect bone by direct osteolysis causing local osteocytic hypercalcemia. Local osteocytic hypercalcemia is due to bony metastases (breast and lung carcinoma most common) or to myeloma which makes factors that stimulate osteoclasts to resorb bone. In 50–80% of patients with malignancy, the hypercalcemia cannot be attributed to tumor invasion of the bone. These patients have humoral hypercalcemia of malignancy. Various tumors (squamous cell carcinomas of any organ, renal cell carcinoma, adenocarcinoma of breast that also causes local osteocytic hypercalcemia, transitional cell carcinoma of bladder, ovarian carcinoma, pheochromocytoma, islet cell carcinoma, and human T cell-associated lymphomas) produce PTH-related peptide. The first 13 amino acids of PTH-related peptide are 70% homologous to the active site of PTH, which accounts for its PTH-like effects. PTH-related peptide is almost always elevated in humoral hypercalcemia of malignancy and undetectable in local osteocytic hypercalcemia and other causes of hypercalcemia. The assay for PTH-related peptide, although not universally available, can be obtained commercially (e.g., PTHRP-IRMA, Nichols). Sample collection requires special tubes to inhibit proteolysis and immediate separation and freezing of serum. Prostaglandin E may be one humoral factor, but prostaglandin synthesis inhibitors such as indomethacin are not very successful in treating humoral hypercalcemia of malignancy. Increased bone resorption by osteoclasts is the common mechanism for hypercalcemia. Ectopic production of PTH by tumor rarely causes this syndrome. Occasionally a patient with lymphoma may have hypercalcemia caused by excessive production of 1,25-dihydroxyvitamin D similar to the granulomatous cells in sarcoidosis discussed below.

Endocrine-Related Hypercalcemia

Thyrotoxicosis is associated with increased bone resorption and increased bone turnover. The hypercalcemia is modest and abates as the hyperthyroidism resolves with treatment. Acute adrenal insufficiency is occasionally associated with hypercalcemia that resolves with glucocorticoid treatment. The mechanism for the hypercalcemia of Addison's disease is not understood. Pheochromocytoma may be associated with hypercalcemia as part of the multiple endocrine neoplasia syndromes. The pheochromocytoma is managed surgically before parathyroid exploration. Familial hypocalciuric hypercalcemia differs from primary hyperparathyroidism in several respects: age, urine calcium, complications, and response to surgery. This is a familial disorder in which most patients present before age 20. Urine calcium excretion is inappropriately low for the degree of hypercalcemia, often less than 100 mg/day (most hyperparathyroid patients excrete >250 mg/day). Complications of hypercalcemia such as nephrolithiasis and peptic ulcer disease are rare. Furthermore, subtotal parathyroidectomy does not cure the hypercalcemia, although total parathyroidectomy causes hypocalcemia. The pathophysiology of this unusual autosomal dominant syndrome is unknown, and management is first to "do no harm." Because complications are rare and surgery does not correct the hypercalcemia, operation is avoided. Effort should be directed toward identification and education of other family members.

Medication-Related Hypercalcemia

Thiazide diuretics and related drugs (e.g., chlorthalidone) are natriuretic but not calciuretic, leading to decreased calcium excretion in most patients. The hypercalcemic effect of thiazides also occurs in anephric patients, indicating that other organs are affected by diuretics as well. The hypercalcemia (usually <11.5 mg/dL) should resolve within 2–3 weeks after discontinuing the medication. If hypercalcemia persists, then primary hyperparathyroidism is the most likely diagnosis. Vitamin D intoxication may be found in health faddists or as a complication of therapy for hypoparathyroidism, renal osteodystrophy, hypophosphatemic rickets, or intestinal malabsorption. It is particularly likely with ergocalciferol, vitamin D2, which is stored in fat depots for months. Treatment consists of discontinuation of vitamin D and calcium supplements, hydration and diuresis (furosemide), and administration of hydrocortisone (100–200 mg/day) or equivalent steroid until the patient is normocalcemic. Vitamin A intoxication may occur with doses above 50,000 U/day. Pharmacologic doses of vitamin A cause osteoclastic bone resorption. Any patient with a skin disorder may be receiving vitamin A, so history is important. The treatment is as for vitamin D intoxication. Milk-alkali syndrome results from ingestion of large amounts of calcium carbonate and calcium bicarbonate usually in the treatment of peptic ulcer disease. This syndrome is unusual today because of the use of nonabsorbable antacids. Renal insufficiency, hypocalciuria, alkalosis, and hyperphosphatemia are invariably present. The pathogenesis of lithium-induced hypercalcemia remains obscure.

Granulomatous Diseases

Sarcoidosis is by far the most common cause of hypercalcemia within this group. About 10% of patients with active sarcoidosis have hypercalcemia, but over 40% have hypercalciuria, often with nephrolithiasis. Patients with sarcoidosis are known to have an increased conversion of 25-hydroxyvitamin D to 1,25-dihydroxyvitamin D. This correlates with the observation that sarcoid patients become hypercalcemic on small doses of vitamin D2 (10,000 U/day), whereas most normal subjects tolerate 10 times this amount without overt hypercalcemia. Hypercalcemia is more prevalent in sarcoidosis during the summer when endogenous production of vitamin D is increased. Serum levels of 1,25-dihydroxyvitamin D are elevated in active sarcoidosis, but the mechanism responsible for this conversion is not yet understood. Treatment with glucocorticoids should be correlated with activity of the underlying granulomatous disease.

Immobilization

Immobilization of patients with Paget's disease or other states of high bone turnover (as in children) is likely to result in hypercalcemia as well as hypercalciuria. Treatment consists of hydration and early ambulation.

HYPOCALCEMIA

Because about half of the total serum calcium is bound to protein, a low serum calcium should be anticipated in cases of low albumin. Acute hyperventilation leads to alkalosis, which lowers ionized calcium without changing total serum calcium. A low serum ionized calcium produces characteristic symptoms. The severity and duration of the hypocalcemia dictate the clinical presentation. Acute hypocalcemia is much more likely to be symptomatic than chronic hypocalcemia despite equivalent levels of serum calcium.

Signs and symptoms of neuromuscular irritability predominate and include weakness, muscle cramps, paresthesia of hands and feet, and tetany. Epileptiform seizures and laryngospasm are common presentations in children. Signs of latent tetany include Chvostek's sign (tapping facial nerve over the parotid elicits a twitch at the angle of the mouth) and Trousseau's sign (inflating the sphygmomanometer about 20 mmHg above the systolic blood pressure for 3 minutes produces carpal spasm—flexion of the wrist and metacarpophalangeal joints and adduction of the thumb). A faint Chvostek's sign is present in about 10% of the normal population, but development of a strong Chvostek's sign after neck surgery suggests hypocalcemia. Trousseau's sign is a more reliable indicator of hypocalcemia. Tetany is not specific for hypocalcemia and may be seen in hypomagnesemia, in hypokalemia, and in respiratory alkalosis as mentioned above. Idiopathic hypoparathyroidism may be associated with mucocutaneous candidiasis. Cataracts are common in chronic hypocalcemia; the cause is unknown, but treatment of the hypocalcemia stops their progression.

Laboratory Studies

Serum calcium is <8.5 mg/dL (provided serum albumin is normal), and ionized calcium is <1.07 mmol/L. Serum phosphate is usually high (>5.0 mg/dL) in hypoparathyroidism and normal to low in vitamin D deficient states. Calcification of the basal ganglia is seen in about half of the children with chronic hypocalcemia and may be associated with extrapyramidal signs of parkinsonism and choreoathetosis.

Causes

The differential diagnosis of hypocalcemia includes hypoparathyroidism caused by PTH deficiency or resistance (pseudohypoparathyroidism); hypomagnesemia; pancreatitis; acute phosphate intoxication; and vitamin D deficiency, malabsorption, and renal insufficiency as discussed in Chapter 13.

Hypoparathyroidism

Deficiency of PTH may be a complication of neck surgery (thyroid, parathyroid, surgery for carcinoma of larynx). Surgical hypoparathyroidism is the most common cause of hypoparathyroidism. Hypocalcemia after surgery for hyperparathyroidism is usually related to the "hungry bone syndrome." These patients have hypophosphatemia as opposed to the typical hyperphosphatemia of true parathyroid deficiency. Management of surgical hypoparathyroidism is generally much easier than idiopathic hypoparathyroidism since smaller doses of vitamin D or even calcium supplements alone correct the hypocalcemia; presumably some PTH is still being produced. Idiopathic hypoparathyroidism is rare and may occur alone or be associated with autoimmune polyglandular failure. Most cases are sporadic and occur before age 15. Hypoparathyroidism is the result of total atrophy of the parathyroid glands. Associated autoimmune diseases include hypoparathyroidism, Addison's disease, and moniliasis (HAM syndrome) as well hypothyroidism, pernicious anemia, ovarian failure, vitiligo, and myasthenia gravis. The diagnosis of hypoparathyroidism is confirmed by measurement of PTH (it is low to nonmeasurable in primary hypoparathyroidism and high in pseudohypoparathyroidism). The hypocalcemia of idiopathic hypoparathyroidism is severe (average total serum calcium is 5.4 mg/dL) and requires full doses of calcium and vitamin D.

Pseudohypoparathyroidism

Pseudohypoparathyroidism is a familial syndrome of hypocalcemia associated with raised levels of PTH and resistance to PTH action. A

characteristic physiognomy (Albright's osteodystrophy) of round facies, short stature, and short metacarpals and metatarsals (fourth and
fifth digits) is present in the classic syndrome. The importance of this
syndrome relates not to its frequency but rather to its contribution to
our understanding of the pathophysiology of hormone resistance in
general. Pseudohypoparathyroidism is managed as hypoparathyroidism but is often easier to treat than idiopathic hypoparathyroidism, probably because hormone resistance is not total. Patients
who have the stigmata of Albright's osteodystrophy (short stature,
obesity, and dystrophic bone changes) without hypocalcemia are said
to have pseudopseudohypoparathyroidism, which is genetically related but distinct from pseudohypoparathyroidism.

Hypomagnesemia

Severe hypomagnesemia (under 0.8 mEq/L) may cause hypocalcemia by inhibiting PTH effect on bone and by decreasing the secretion of PTH by the parathyroid gland in response to hypocalcemia.
This syndrome is found in chronic alcoholism and malabsorption.
The hypocalcemia fails to respond to calcium loading but is relieved
by magnesium replacement (page 41).

Other Causes of Hypocalcemia

Pancreatitis may cause a transitory hypocalcemia. The mechanism remains unexplained. Vitamin D deficiency and disorders of vitamin D
metabolism as causes of hypocalcemia are discussed in Chapter 13
under "Osteomalacia."

Treatment

Chronic hypocalcemia is treated with calcium supplementation and
with vitamin D or one of its analogs. Doses in the range of 1.5–2.0 g
elemental calcium/day are prescribed in three divided doses daily
usually at meals. Calcium content of the available preparations varies,
so verify that the proper amount of elemental calcium is taken.
Calcium carbonate, the most convenient and most economical form,
has the highest calcium content (40%), which means fewer tablets are
needed. Calcium chloride should be avoided because of the high incidence of gastric irritation. Table 12.2 lists several calcium preparations, their calcium content, and approximate cost per day for 1.5 g
elemental calcium.

Table 12.2
Calcium Preparations Used to Treat Chronic Hypocalcemia

Compound	Trade Name	Calcium Content (mg)	Tablets/Day	Cost/Day[a]
Calcium carbonate	Generic 500	500	3	7–10¢
	OsCal 500	500	3	35–40¢
	Titralac (420 mg)	168	9	55–75¢
	Tums	200	8	30–40¢
Calcium lactate	Generic (625 mg)	80	19	50–75¢
Calcium gluconate	Generic (1 g)	90	17	$1.60
Calcium glubionate	Neo-Calglucon (5 mL)	115	4 tbsp	$1.85

[a]Approximate cost to patient for 1.5 g elemental calcium if 100 tablets purchased.

Vitamin D and its analogs promote intestinal absorption of calcium. The preparation and dose of vitamin D vary depending on the underlying cause of the hypocalcemia. Vitamin D2 (ergocalciferol) is the traditional preparation. Its principal advantage is low cost, an important factor because this is a lifetime medication for most patients. The disadvantage of vitamin D2 is that the therapeutic dose is close to the toxic dose and, thus, may cause hypercalcemia. Because this vitamin is stored in fat, it may take up to 3 months for any hypercalcemia to resolve. The onset of action likewise is delayed and may take up to 1–2 months to achieve maximal effect. Large doses (ergocalciferol 50,000–100,000 U/day) are needed for most hypocalcemic disorders in order to override the decreased activity of kidney hydroxylase caused by the lack of PTH. Despite these drawbacks, most patients can be managed successfully with this preparation. Care is taken to check the serum calcium every 3–6 months since some patients who appear to be under optimal control will unexpectedly develop hypercalcemia. Remember that hypoparathyroid patients lack the renal effects of PTH; one significant action is to increase tubular resorption of calcium. Thus, at any serum level of calcium, the kidneys waste calcium, making hypercalciuria possible even though serum calcium is not elevated. Measuring urine calcium while on treatment enables one to avoid hypercalciuria that might lead to renal stones and nephrocalcinosis. Smaller doses of ergocalciferol are used to treat vitamin D deficiency (5000 U/day initially, then 400 U/day) and for the anticonvulsant therapy-related hypocalcemia (5000 U/day). Dihydrotachysterol is another vitamin D preparation used in the treatment of chronic hypocalcemia. It is a synthetic analog of vitamin D that does not require 1-α-hydroxylation by the kidney. The potency of dihydrotachysterol is not as great nor the onset of action as short as the latest vitamin D preparation, 1,25-dihydroxyvitamin D (calcitriol). Calcitriol has the advantages of a rapid onset of action (2–4 days) and a short half-life (12–24 hours); the latter allows quick resolution should the complication of hypercalcemia arise. Both dihydrotachysterol and calcitriol offer the theoretical advantage of circumventing the need for renal hydroxylation that is impaired in PTH deficiency and PTH resistance. Cost is the major disadvantage of long-term calcitriol therapy. For the patient who does not reliably take their medications, ergocalciferol is preferable to calciferol. Calcidiol (25-hydroxyvitamin D) offers no advantages in the treatment of hypocalcemia. Table 12.3 lists the preparations of vitamin D and its derivatives.

Table 12.3
Vitamin D Preparations Used to Treat Hypocalcemia

Drug	Trade Name	Daily Dose	Cost/Day[a]
Ergocalciferol	Drisdol	50,000–100,000 U	40–80¢
Dihydrotachysterol	Hytakerol	125–250 µg	$2.00–3.00
25-Hydroxyvitamin D	Calderol	50–100 µg[b]	$2.20–4.40
1,25-Dihydroxyvitamin D	Rocaltrol	0.25–1.0 µg[b]	$1.60–3.20

[a]Cost to patient when 100 tablets purchased, markup may vary.
[b]Often taken twice a day.

Regardless of the preparation chosen, close monitoring of the serum calcium is mandatory, usually weekly until eucalcemia is obtained, then every 3–6 months. If hypercalciuria develops, then reduce dose of calcium and/or vitamin D supplementation. Those patients with chronic hypocalcemia replacement must wear proper identification regarding their medical diagnosis and medications (e.g., Medic-Alert).

Suggested Readings

Audran M, Kumar R: The physiology and pathophysiology of vitamin D. *Mayo Clin Proc* 60:851, 1985.

Barzel US: Primary hyperparathyroidism: problems in management. *Hosp Pract* 27:165, 1992.

Bilezikian JP: Primary hyperparathyroidism. In Bardin CW (ed): *Current Therapy in Endocrinology and Metabolism*, ed 4. Philadelphia, Decker, 1991, pp 448–452.

Chapman I, Horowitz M, Need AG, Morris HA: Primary hyperparathyroidism: pathogenesis, diagnosis, and management. *Compr Ther* 14:65, 1988.

Marx SJ, Speigel AM, Brown EM, et al: Divalent cation metabolism. Familial hypocalciuric hypercalcemia versus typical primary hyperparathyroidism. *Am J Med* 65:235, 1978.

Patten BM, Bilezikian JP, Mallette LE, Prince A, Engel WK, Aurbach GD: Neuromuscular disease in primary hyperparathyroidism. *Ann Intern Med* 80:182, 1974.

Stewart AF, Broadus AE: Mineral metabolism. In Felig P, Baxter JD, Broadus AE, Frohman LA (eds): *Endocrinology and Metabolism*, ed 2. New York, McGraw-Hill, 1986, pp 1317–1453.

Wang C, Gaz RD: Natural history of parathyroid carcinoma: diagnosis, treatment, and results. *Am J Surg* 149:522, 1985.

Chapter 13

Metabolic Bone Disease

Metabolic bone disease refers to various disorders that affect bony tissue including <u>osteoporosis</u>, <u>osteomalacia</u>, <u>osteitis fibrosa</u>, <u>renal osteodystrophy</u>, and <u>osteitis deformans (Paget's disease of bone)</u>. Bone is a dynamic tissue that is constantly undergoing change. Remodeling at bone surfaces is a complex process involving matrix (osteoid) synthesis by osteoblasts, mineralization of the matrix to form mature bone, and eventually resorption of calcified bone by osteoclasts. The process that results in mineralization of the osteoid is poorly understood, but proper amounts of calcium, phosphate, vitamin D metabolites, and a normal collagen matrix are necessary for this process to proceed normally. In addition, <u>local</u> factors such as mechanical stress and coupling factors (proteins that link resorption with formation and vice versa) are involved in the remodeling process. Because bone formation and bone resorption are processes that can be modified by the hormone and chemical milieu, various different disorders may lead to metabolic bone disease.

OSTEOPOROSIS

Osteoporosis, the most common metabolic bone disease, is an important cause of morbidity and mortality for the elderly. Osteoporotic bone has decreased bone volume (less mineralized matrix per unit volume) and less trabecular bridging, leading to fewer struts for support. The bone matrix appears to mineralize normally. Osteoporosis affects all bone, but trabecular bone (e.g., vertebrae, femoral head, distal radius) is much more involved than compact or cortical bone (e.g., shafts of long bones). Reduced mass in trabecular bones means that these affected bones are subject to collapse and fracture. The osteo-

porotic patient usually presents with compression fractures of spinal
vertebral bodies or fractures of distal radius or proximal femur.

The pathogenesis of osteoporosis is multifactorial. Bone mineral
content reaches its maximum during the third decade of life. The
amount of mineral deposited depends on body size (thin, petite-
framed have less mineral than large-framed individuals), sex (females
have less than males), and race (Caucasians have less than Negroes).
After the third decade there is a gradual reduction in body mineral
content that is accelerated in the menopausal female. Estrogen is vital
in preservation of mineral mass. Estrogen deficiency is associated with
lower serum levels of 1,25-dihydroxyvitamin D that lead to less intestinal absorption of calcium. Estrogen also inhibits parathyroid hormone (PTH) effect on bone resorption. These factors plus an inadequate dietary intake of calcium by most adult women and possibly less
sunlight exposure are thought to be the reasons for the acceleration of
mineral loss from the bone. Bone biopsy of osteoporotic patients confirms a multifactorial causation since some patients have increased
bone resorption as well as decreased bone formation. Table 13.1 lists
the risk factors for osteoporosis.

The risk factor that most reliably identifies individuals subject to
osteoporosis is low bone mass. The reduced mineral content can be
demonstrated as osteopenia on roentgenographs (only after there has
been a >30% decrease in trabecular bone mass) and by bone absorptiometry. Bone mineral content can be measured with reasonable accuracy and reproducibility. Single photon absorptiometry assesses
mineral content at the os calcis and midshaft and distal radius. Dual

Table 13.1
Risk Factors for Osteoporosis in Women

White or Oriental race
Petite frame
Inadequate dietary intake of calcium
Early menopause or oophorectomy
Positive family history for osteoporosis
Alcohol abuse
Cigarette smoking
Sedentary lifestyle
Reduced bone mineral content
    (most predictive risk factor)

photon absorptiometry and dual-energy X-ray absorptiometry measure bone mass at the spine and hip; scan time and radiation dose are much less with the latter method.

Osteoporosis has always been difficult to categorize because of its insidious onset. Postmenopausal or Type I osteoporosis occurs in women aged 51–65 years presenting with vertebral fractures. Senile osteoporosis or Type II osteoporosis affects both men and women older than age 70 and involves fractures of both cortical and trabecular bone. There are several endocrine abnormalities associated with osteoporosis. These include estrogen deficiency during the premenopausal years as in ovarian dysgenesis (Turner's syndrome) or premature menopause (surgical or idiopathic); testosterone deficiency; Cushing's syndrome; hyperthyroidism; and primary hyperparathyroidism. Whether diabetes mellitus increases the risk of osteoporosis is controversial. Immobilization or weightlessness can also cause osteoporosis.

The clinical presentation of osteoporosis is pain and deformity related to fracture. Back pain is usually the symptom that brings the patient to the physician. Onset of pain may be sudden, aggravated by movement and weight bearing, and relieved by rest. Thoracic and lumbar vertebrae are most affected (especially T12 and L1). Falling is particularly likely to lead to femoral neck fractures or Colles' fracture of the wrist (both areas of considerable trabecular bone). Lost of vertebral height and anterior wedging of the vertebrae lead to shortening of stature and kyphosis.

Laboratory Studies

Laboratory findings are usually *not* diagnostic, with serum calcium, phosphorus, and alkaline phosphatase activity being normal. The X-ray often shows generalized osteopenia as well as the site of fracture. Ballooning of nuclei pulposi into weakened trabecular bone leads to concave deformities ("codfishing") of the vertebra, and localized herniation of the pulposus leads to Schmorl's node. Radiographs are notoriously poor in judging bone mass, so measuring bone mineral content identifies bone mass below fracture threshold.

If there is no osteopenia or decreased bone mineral content or if there are serum calcium or phosphatase abnormalities in a female who presents with a compression vertebral fracture, one should consider the possibility of a pathological fracture caused by metastatic disease. If there are anemia and vertebral fractures, myeloma should be excluded.

Therapy

Treatment of newly diagnosed vertebral fractures includes <u>bed rest</u>, <u>analgesics for pain</u>, and <u>local heat for relief of paravertebral muscle spasm</u> that often develops as the major component of chronic back pain. Avoid using narcotics for analgesia if possible. <u>Early ambulation is recommended.</u> If pain persists, back support in the form of a back brace is used. Patients are cautioned not to lift heavy objects and to bend at the knees instead of the waist when lifting objects. Exercise such as long walks is encouraged. Finally, therapy should be directed toward preventing falls and arresting further bone loss. Many fractures occur after falls at home. Encourage patients to use props (aids to locomotion, walkers, canes, rails on both sides of stairwells, walls), remove throw rugs and other hazards, and use night lights.

Unfortunately there are no drugs that provoke or increase the amount of <u>normal</u> bone mass. At present, all medications are given <u>to retard</u> progression of the loss of mineral mass that accompanies aging. It is difficult to evaluate whether a treatment regimen is suitable or is working in an individual unless one uses bone mineral content obtained by absorptiometry. Photon absorption of the radius tells little about the axial skeleton where loss of mineral is the greatest. Various noninvasive studies such as dual photon absorptiometry (cost $200) and computed tomography of the vertebral body (cost $700) are useful to follow the effectiveness of the treatment regimen. Most recommended treatments are derived from epidemiologic studies of populations of patients treated with different regimens.

The safest medication is <u>calcium supplementation</u>—1.0–1.5 g elemental calcium/day taken as calcium carbonate for convenience (page 170). Oral calcium ingestion corrects any negative calcium balance and inhibits bone loss via resorption. Its overall effectiveness is difficult to discern.

<u>Estrogen</u> is effective in treating osteoporosis. It retards bone loss by inhibiting PTH-induced resorption and by increasing gut absorption of calcium. Estrogen therapy has been demonstrated to reduce the fracture rate in osteoporosis, to reduce the loss of height, and to retard mineral loss from vertebral bodies. Estrogen treatment produces its best effect in the perimenopausal years. At least 0.625 mg conjugated equine estrogens or 1.0 mg micronized estradiol is necessary to be effective. However, estrogens have troublesome side effects including vaginal bleeding, increased risk of endometrial carcinoma, and tendency to fluid retention. Sequential estrogen-progestin or con-

current daily estrogen-progestin can be prescribed (page 111). Women who have had a hysterectomy need only take estrogen. Annual breast examinations are necessary, and all abnormal vaginal bleeding must be promptly investigated. <u>The ideal candidate for estrogen therapy is the woman who has had a hysterectomy.</u>

<u>Vitamin D</u> is not used alone for therapy. Providing most patients with small doses of vitamin D2 (400 U/day) is sufficient to meet vitamin D requirements. High doses of vitamin D2 (Drisdal 50,000 U twice a week) can lead to hypercalciuria and possibly to hypercalcemia. However, pharmacological doses of vitamin D are used for patients with impaired bowel absorption of calcium. Generally these patients have <50 mg urine calcium/24 hour (normal 150–250 mg/day). These patients may well have osteomalacia in addition to osteoporosis on bone biopsy.

<u>Calcitonin</u> increases total body calcium. Calcitonin helps the pain around the interval of acute and subacute fracture. Patients who cannot take estrogen (e.g., history of breast cancer) or have "high" turnover osteoporosis (increased biochemical parameters of resorption) are good candidates for calcitonin therapy. Widespread use has not occurred because of poor patient compliance, cost, and route of administration (subcutaneous or intramuscular daily to twice weekly).

<u>Bisphosphonates</u>, such as etidronate, inhibit bone resorption by coating the mineral surfaces such that the osteoclasts cannot hydrolyze the mineral as well as some direct effect on the osteoclasts. Short-term studies suggest beneficial effect with fewer fractures, but whether biphosphonates prevent hip fractures and long-term vertebral fractures is unknown.

<u>Fluoride</u> increases bone mass, but the bone is *not* normal. The doses used, 40–60 mg/day, may cause gastric irritation and bleeding, osteomalacia, and secondary hyperparathyroidism. Fluoride therapy is still experimental and is *not* approved for use by the Food and Drug Administration for treatment of osteoporosis.

Preventive Treatment

Preventive therapy begins by encouraging adequate calcium and exercise for all ages, treating hypogonadism of premenopausal females, avoiding over-replacing hypothyroid patients with thyroxine, and identifying those at increased risk for osteoporosis. Patients are asked to ingest oral calcium 1.0–1.5 g and 400 U vitamin D daily. Most menopausal women should be prescribed estrogen not only to retard bone loss but for the protective cardiovascular effects of estrogen. Despite the almost universal recommendation for estrogen supplementation, many women do not take them. For those concerned women who question the value of estrogen, measurement of bone density with the finding of bone mineral content 80% below the mean for age-matched controls may provide impetus for a change of mind. Foster exercise and use immobilization only for the acute situation. Again, any aids that prevent falls, the cause of most hip and Colles' fractures, are to be encouraged. Smoking and alcohol abuse should be discouraged. If the osteoporosis is related to glucocorticoid excess, then reduction of steroid if possible is indicated along with oral calcium, vitamin D, and/or calcitonin.

OSTEOMALACIA

Osteomalacia is characterized by <u>large amounts of osteoid that do not mineralize</u>. Bone mineralization depends on adequate concentrations of calcium and phosphorus locally along the surface of normal bone matrix. If the matrix is not mineralized progressively, then large amounts of osteoid accumulate because of the continual formation of matrix by osteoblasts. Again the inter-relationships among calcium, phosphate, vitamin D and its metabolites, and PTH are important for mineralization of bone. <u>Any disorder that lowers serum calcium or decreases serum phosphate can lead to osteomalacia.</u>

The clinical presentation of osteomalacia <u>depends on age and severity and duration of the underlying disorder</u>. In children osteomalacia is called rickets. Rickets causes <u>deformity</u> in areas of bone that are most rapidly growing, leading to craniotabes, frontal bossing, enlargement of costochondral junctions ("rachitic rosary"), and bowing of the legs. Large areas of unmineralized and disorganized epiphyseal growth-plate cartilage lead to short stature. In adult-onset rickets (osteomalacia) bone deformity is rare. What are common in both rickets and osteomalacia are <u>bone pain</u> and <u>local tenderness</u> over severely affected areas. Muscle weakness is common, particularly in the proximal muscles of the lower extremities. If the patient is also hypocalcemic, paresthesia, tetany, and seizures may be present.

The radiographic picture of advanced childhood rickets is quite characteristic: enlargement of unmineralized epiphyseal growth plates; widening and cupping associated with a frayed appearance of the metaphyses; and pseudofractures. In adults, osteomalacia often appears as <u>generalized osteopenia</u> mimicking osteoporosis and making radiographic distinction difficult. A characteristic radiographic feature pathognomonic for osteomalacia is the <u>pseudofracture</u> (Looser's zones or Milkman fractures). Pseudofractures are most often bilateral and occur in the femoral neck and shaft, ulna and radius, clavicle, scapula, pubic and ischial rami, and small bones of the hands and feet. Secondary hyperparathyroidism, found in vitamin D deficiency osteomalacia, causes bone resorption manifested by subperiosteal resorption of phalanges, loss of lamina dura of the teeth, resorption of the distal clavicle, widening of the pubic symphysis and the sacroiliac joint space, and bone cysts or brown tumors (see "Osteitis Fibrosa").

Osteomalacia can be classified biochemically into two subgroups. (*a*) The result of <u>vitamin D deficiency or altered vitamin D metabolism</u> leading to inadequate calcium absorption from the gut and <u>low serum calcium</u>. Secondary hyperparathyroidism results from the attempt to normalize serum calcium and leads to <u>lowering of the serum phosphorus</u> as a result of PTH-induced phosphaturia. <u>Serum alkaline phosphatase activity is elevated</u> by osteoblastic activation coupled to bone resorption effects of PTH. (*b*) A <u>defect in phosphate transport</u> leading to phosphaturia and poor gut absorption of phosphorus manifested by <u>normocalcemia</u> and severe <u>hypophosphatemia</u>. The serum alkaline phosphatase activity is also increased. There is no evidence of hyperparathyroidism in this chronic hypophosphatemic group.

Assays of vitamin D and its metabolites have been helpful in assessing the heterogeneous causes of osteomalacia. Vitamin D is a prohormone that is eaten in the diet or derived from the conversion of a steroid in the skin to vitamin D by sunlight (ultraviolet spectrum). Vitamin D itself has little, if any, biological activity, but it is hydroxylated by a liver enzyme, vitamin D 25-hydroxylase, leading to the major vitamin D metabolite in the serum, 25-hydroxyvitamin D. <u>Measurement of serum 25-hydroxyvitamin D is the best indicator of body stores of vitamin D; it is low in vitamin D deficiency states</u> (normal ranges are 8–60 ng/mL). The most active metabolite of vitamin D is <u>1,25-dihydroxyvitamin D</u>, which is derived from further hydroxylation of 25-hydroxyvitamin D in the kidney. Elevated PTH levels and low serum phosphorus stimulate the formation of 1,25-dihydroxyvitamin D. Low levels of PTH and high serum phosphorus will lower the level of this metabolite. Normal serum 1,25-dihydroxyvitamin D ranges between 20 and 50 pg/mL.

Regardless of the causal biochemical defect, the <u>clinical and radiographic presentation of osteomalacia is constant</u>. However, the biochemical defect is helpful in determining the etiology of the osteomalacia and in selecting the most effective therapy. As mentioned above, osteomalacia is classified on the basis of abnormalities related to vitamin D or to chronic hypophosphatemia.

Abnormal Vitamin D Metabolism

Vitamin D abnormalities include reduced circulating vitamin D metabolites (because of <u>inadequate sunlight exposure</u>, <u>inadequate dietary vitamin D</u>, <u>vitamin D malabsorption</u> as a result of small intestine disease, bile salt, or pancreatic insufficiency) and <u>abnormal vitamin D metabolism</u> (caused by liver disease, chronic renal failure, drugs such as phenytoin and phenobarbital that decrease 25-hydroxyvitamin D levels, mesenchymal tumors and prostatic carcinoma that are associated with low 1,25-dihydroxyvitamin D levels, vitamin D-dependent rickets Type I where the renal 1-α-hydroxylase activity is very low). Resistance to 1,25-dihydroxyvitamin D is rare and is called vitamin D-dependent rickets Type II.

Vitamin D-related osteomalacia has usually been treated with vitamin D2, the plant-derived vitamin, which is inexpensive. Large enough doses can override many of the above defects by mass action. For prevention of vitamin D deficiency 100 IU/day is sufficient in adults and 400 IU/day for children. Pharmacological doses up to 100,000 IU vitamin D2/day are needed in bowel malabsorption osteomalacia. Patients with gluten enteropathy resolve their osteomalacia with a gluten-free diet alone. Patients taking anticonvulsant therapy need 5000 IU vitamin D2/day to treat and prevent osteomalacia. Patients with chronic renal failure and vitamin D-resistant rickets Type I respond to physiological amounts of 1,25-dihydroxyvitamin D (0.5–2.0 μg/day).

Each vitamin D preparation has advantages and disadvantages. Vitamin D2 is cheap and usually effective, but the therapeutic dose approaches the toxic dose, onset of action is slow (weeks), and duration is prolonged because this vitamin is stored in fat. Other preparations are available (25-hydroxyvitamin D and dihydrotachysterol), but these are relatively expensive and offer no real practical advantages. Calcitriol (1,25-dihydroxyvitamin D; Rocaltrol) is expensive ($80–100/100 0.25-μg tablets), but onset of action is rapid (2–4 days) and half-life short (12 hours). Because calcitriol is the active compound, no transformation is needed to make it active.

Hypophosphatemic Rickets

<u>Hypophosphatemic vitamin D-resistant rickets</u> is the most common form of osteomalacia in the United States. <u>Renal phosphate wasting</u> (phosphate diabetes) is the cardinal feature. PTH does not contribute to the phosphaturia. Familial X-linked hypophosphatemic rickets is another name for this syndrome, but the pattern of inheritance is not well established because sporadic and autosomal recessive patterns have been reported. Other maladies associated with significant phosphaturia include Fanconi's syndrome and tumor-induced osteomalacia. Chronic hypophosphatemia secondary to phosphate binding antacids may rarely lead to osteomalacia.

Hypophosphatemic vitamin D-resistant rickets is treated with oral phosphate (elemental phosphorus 1–4 g/day) given in divided doses to minimize diarrhea. Although oral phosphate may raise the serum phosphorus and improve the osteomalacia as assessed by roentgenographs, complete bone healing is seen only in patients treated with phosphates *and* 1,25-dihydroxyvitamin D, 1–3 μg/day.

OSTEITIS FIBROSA

Osteitis fibrosa is characterized by resorption of bone, osteoclastic activation with focal eroded areas (Howship's lacunae), reactive fibrosis, cyst formation, and brown tumors. <u>Hyperparathyroidism</u> is the underlying biochemical defect causing bone resorption and subsequent <u>hypercalcemia</u>. 1,25-Dihydroxyvitamin D levels are usually elevated because PTH stimulates renal synthesis of this metabolite. As a result of coupling reaction in bone, osteoblasts are activated, leading to <u>raised levels of alkaline phosphatase activity</u>. Secondary hyperparathyroidism, as in chronic renal failure, may lead to osteitis fibrosa.

The radiographic changes associated with hyperparathyroidism reflect bone resorption: osteopenia; subperiosteal resorption of phalanges (especially lateral midshaft) and clavicles (particularly lateral ends); and small punched-out lesions of the skull. Osteitis fibrosa cystica represents a late effect of chronic hyperparathyroidism. These classic bone changes are seen less frequently than in the past because hypercalcemia is often found with screening chemistries.

The treatment of primary hyperparathyroidism is generally with surgery. Removal of the abnormal parathyroid gland(s) is the only effective therapy. Estrogens block the effect of PTH on bone and should be considered second-line treatment. Postoperative hypocalcemia after parathyroid surgery should be anticipated owing to the "hungry bone" and treated with oral or intravenous calcium.

RENAL OSTEODYSTROPHY

Renal osteodystrophy is the metabolic bone disease that accompanies chronic renal insufficiency and failure. The combination of <u>hyperphosphatemia</u> (inhibits 1,25-dihydroxyvitamin D synthesis) and loss of renal mass (decreased 25-hydroxyvitamin D 1-α-hydroxylase) reduces the active D metabolite leading to calcium malabsorption and consequent <u>hypocalcemia</u>. Hypocalcemia leads to osteomalacia as well as secondary hyperparathyroidism. The bone lesions of renal osteodystrophy are highly variable and may reflect osteomalacia, osteitis fibrosa, or both. Pain, weakness, and fractures are common with this disorder.

The best treatment is prevention because most, if not all, patients with chronic azotemia develop some form of renal osteodystrophy. <u>Maintenance of normal serum calcium and phosphorus concentrations</u> is the first goal. Restricting dietary phosphorus to 1 g/day, using phosphate-binding antacids, providing at least 1–1.5 g elemental calcium/day, and maintaining acid balance with judicious use of alkali are important therapeutic points in prevention of renal osteodystrophy. Prophylactic use of calcitriol is useful, but close follow-up is needed to avoid hypercalcemia and extraskeletal calcification. Bone biopsy after tetracycline labeling of the mineralization front (a technique available in centers that evaluate bone histomorphology with ultraviolet microscopy) is helpful in patients with advanced bone disease to assess whether there is low turnover osteomalacia, aggressive osteitis fibrosa, or any combination thereof. Selective partial parathyroidectomy may be necessary for osteitis fibrosa.

PAGET'S DISEASE OF THE BONE

Paget's disease (osteitis deformans) is a chronic, patchy, and scattered disease affecting localized areas of bone. It is common in up to 4% of the population with an Anglo-Saxon origin older than 40. The etiology is unknown. The disease may affect one or multiple areas of bone (polyostotic form). The areas of affected bone are characterized by <u>localized osteolysis with giant osteoclasts containing up to 100 nuclei</u>. The number of nuclei within the pagetic osteoclast is much greater than in other metabolic bone diseases. In addition, large numbers of osteoblasts are present, forming bone in areas of previous osteolytic activity. Unfortunately this bone structure and modeling is not normal. If severe, these lesions lead to bone deformity and enlargement. Inclusions that have the appearance of viral nucleocapsids have been identified and have raised again the view of Sir James Paget that this disease is inflammatory in nature.

Clinical features are variable. Most patients are <u>asymptomatic</u>, and the disorder is discovered as the result of screening chemistries. <u>The serum alkaline phosphatase activity is elevated, and the serum calcium and phosphorus are normal.</u> Chance finding of lytic and sclerotic areas of bone with bone expansion on radiographic examinations is also a frequent method of detecting asymptomatic disease.

Pain and deformity are the most common symptoms. However, bone pain does not correlate well with the degree of skeletal involvement. Nerve root compression (e.g., acoustic nerve), spinal cord or brainstem compression caused by expansive bone, and pathological fractures in weight-bearing bones are the most severe complications. With the great degree of resorptive and osteoblastic activity, blood flow to the affected bones is greatly increased, leading to increased warmth over these areas. When more than one-third of the skeleton is involved, then high output heart failure is possible. The pelvic bone is most frequently involved, followed by the femur, skull, tibia, and spine. Lytic and sclerotic areas of bone with bone expansion are seen on roentgenographs. Occult disease not seen on routine X-rays may be demonstrated with radionuclide bone scans.

<u>No treatment is needed for the asymptomatic patient.</u> Non-narcotic analgesics will relieve most affected patients. In those with <u>unrelieved pain or those with the complications</u> mentioned above, treatment with either <u>calcitonin</u> or <u>diphosphonates</u> is indicated. The decision regarding when to institute therapy and which agent to use requires clinical discernment. Because these agents have been used for only a decade, pros and cons are still evolving.

<u>Calcitonin</u> inhibits bone resorption. Subcutaneous salmon calcitonin 50–100 U is given daily until symptoms improve (usually 2–6 weeks later). Remember to skin test with calcitonin initially since anaphylactic reactions have occasionally been reported. Thereafter, calcitonin is given three times per week and continued for an undefined period (average 22 months). Alkaline phosphatase activity decreases by 50% after 3 months. Calcitonin is relatively expensive, and antibodies to this agent often develop, with up to one-fourth of the patients becoming resistant to salmon calcitonin after an initial biochemical remission.

Table 13.2
Summary of Biochemical Data in Metabolic Bone Disease

Bone Disorder	Serum Calcium	Serum Phosphorus	Alkaline Phosphatase	Urine Calcium
Osteoporosis	Normal	Normal	Normal	Normal[a]
Osteomalacia	Low[b]	Very low	High	Low
Osteitis fibrosa	High	Low	High	High
Renal osteodystrophy	Low	High	High	Low
Paget's disease	Normal	Normal	Very high	Normal

[a] Usually normal but may be high with immobilization or low with poor calcium intake.
[b] Low in vitamin D abnormalities but low normal in chronic hypophosphatemic rickets.

Diphosphonates inhibit both bone resorption and mineralization. Disodium etidronate (Didronil) 5 mg/kg is taken orally daily. Larger doses may be needed, but the risks of mineralization defect (osteomalacia) are greater. The clinical and biochemical response is similar to calcitonin with a few notable exceptions; there is a paradoxical increase in pain in 10% of the patients treated with diphosphonates, and radiographic evidence of healing is seldom seen after diphosphonate therapy. Six months of therapy are often followed by a prolonged biochemical remission (1 or more years). If symptoms recur, another 6-month course can be instituted.

Hypercalcemia is generally not seen in ambulatory patients with Paget's disease. However, hypercalcemia may be a considerable problem in the immobilized pagetic patient, thereby emphasizing the importance of ambulation and adequate hydration in these patients.

Biochemical data for these metabolic bone diseases are reviewed in Table 13.2.

Suggested Readings

Bell NH: Acquired osteomalacia. In Bardin CW (ed): *Current Therapy in Endocrinology and Metabolism,* ed 4. Philadelphia, Decker, 1991, pp 428–432.

Hahn TJ: Drug-induced disorders of vitamin D and mineral metabolism. *J Clin Endocrinol Metab* 9:107, 1980.

Raisz LG: Therapeutic options for the patient with osteoporosis. *Endocrinologist* 1:11, 1991.

Singer FR: Metabolic bone disease. In Felig P, Baxter JD, Broadus AE, Frohman LA (eds): *Endocrinology and Metabolism,* ed 2. New York, McGraw-Hill, 1986, pp 1454–1499.

Chapter 14

Adrenal Disease

Disorders of the adrenal glands are uncommon. However, many classic symptoms and signs of adrenal diseases mimic those of some common medical disorders such as hypertension, obesity, anxiety, depression, and diabetes mellitus. Thus, adrenal disorders are frequently considered whenever these conditions are encountered because correction of any underlying adrenal disease often cures the "common" medical disorder.

The adrenal cortex secretes cortisol (the principal glucocorticoid), aldosterone (the primary mineralocorticoid), and dehydroeipandrosterone and androstenedione (the predominant androgens). The adrenal medulla secretes the catecholamines epinephrine and norepinephrine. Disorders of these adrenal hormones are discussed in the following section.

CUSHING'S SYNDROME

Cushing's syndrome results from glucocorticoid excess. The most common cause of Cushing's syndrome is the use of pharmacological doses of potent glucocorticoids for nonendocrine disorders. Endogenous causes of Cushing's syndrome include (a) Cushing's disease (pituitary-dependent adrenal hyperplasia), which represents 70–80% of all cases of Cushing's syndrome; (b) ectopic adrenocorticotropin (ACTH) syndrome (ACTH secreted by nonpituitary tumors); (c) adrenal tumors (adenoma or carcinoma); and (d) rarely primary adrenal dysplastic disorders such as pigmented micronodular hyperplasia or macronodular hyperplasia. Pigmented micronodular hyperplasia is a familial disorder presenting in childhood or early adulthood with Cushing's syndrome. Some of these patients have immunoglobulins that bind to adrenal ACTH receptors, stimulating adrenosteroidogenesis (similar to hyperthyroidism in Graves' disease). Macronodular adrenal hyper-

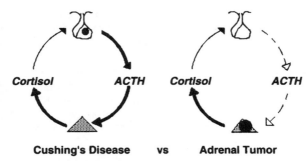

Cushing's Disease   vs   Adrenal Tumor

Figure 14.1. Cushing's syndrome. Two causes of hypercortisolism, pituitary-dependent adrenal hyperplasia and adrenal tumor, are illustrated. A third cause is ectopic ACTH production by various tumors.

plasia, another unusual cause of Cushing's syndrome, is characterized by large adrenal glands with nodular changes. The cause is unknown, but one such patient had cortisol levels that rose in response to food. In this patient gastric inhibitory polypeptide stimulated cortisol production in vivo and in vitro. Figure 14.1 diagrams two causes of hypercortisolism.

Clinical Presentation

The clinical manifestations of glucocorticoid excess are due to the combined effect of glucocorticoids, mineralocorticoids, and adrenal androgens and are identical regardless of its source except for ectopic ACTH syndrome, which usually has few of the chronic changes induced by excess glucocorticoids (e.g., obesity, osteoporosis, etc.) and more of the biochemical changes associated with high doses of corticoids (e.g., hypokalemia and metabolic alkalosis).

Obesity is the most common feature, with the deposition of adipose tissue in the face (round facies), under the chin (dewlap), in supraclavicular fat pads, over the posterior neck, and over the trunk and abdomen. This gives a characteristic physique, i.e., truncal obesity. This centripetal obesity is accentuated by wasting of the extremities caused by the catabolic effect of excess glucocorticoids on muscle. The skin is thin and paper-like, producing facial plethora and less frequently violaceous striae. Protein catabolism leads to muscle weakness, back pain caused by osteoporosis, and easy bruising. Hypertension is virtually universal in patients older than 40 years (reflecting excess mineralocorticoid activity) but is much less common in younger patients. Mild hirsutism, menstrual disorders, and acne are the result of excess adrenal androgens. Psychological disturbances are present in two-thirds of Cushing's patients and may be dramatic with severe depression, psychosis, or mania. Some patients note polyuria that might be due to cortisol-induced suppression of antidiuretic hormone or to frank hyperglycemia in 10–15% of patients. Hypokalemia and metabolic alkalosis are characteristic of ectopic ACTH syndrome.

Workup

The general appearance of the patient often leads one to suspect glucocorticoid excess. Serial photographs taken months and years earlier are most informative (start with driver's license or employment photo). Is the patient taking medication? Always search for a pharmaceutical source of steroids. Is the patient female? Cushing's disease is nine times more common in females than males. Ectopic ACTH syndrome occurs with equal frequency between sexes. How old is the patient? Cushing's disease is most frequent between ages 20 and 40 years. Ectopic ACTH syndrome is generally a disease of the older population. Is there weight loss to suggest ectopic ACTH? Oat cell carcinoma of the lung causes at least half the cases of ectopic ACTH production. Other tumors that secrete ACTH include pancreatic islet cell carcinoma, thymoma, carcinoid tumors, medullary thyroid carcinoma, and pheochromocytoma.

Laboratory

A 24-hour urine for free cortisol and/or 17-hydroxycorticosteroids should be collected in all suspected cases. Always measure urine creatinine to assure adequacy of collection. Although an overnight dexamethasone test can be used to screen for hypercortisolism (page 14), the urine study is more accurate and less likely to give false-positive results. If the urine free cortisol is increased, ACTH determinations should be obtained. High levels are found in ectopic ACTH syndromes (>400 pg/mL), and nonmeasurable ACTH levels (<5 pg/mL) are found in primary adrenal tumors and/or nodular dysplasia. If two ACTH levels are low, then proceed with the abdominal computed tomography (CT); if ACTH levels are normal or high, then perform the Liddle suppression study (page 15). Given clear instructions, most patients can reliably undergo this study as outpatients. Other studies are helpful. Hypokalemia and metabolic alkalosis in the absence of diuretic therapy suggest ectopic ACTH as does a chest X-ray that demonstrates a mass lesion. Very elevated urinary 17-ketosteroids (higher than the urinary 17-hydroxycorticosteroid) suggest adrenal carcinoma.

Adrenal tumors can be identified with the high resolution adrenal CT scan. Unfortunately the CT and magnetic resonance imaging scans of the pituitary are not diagnostic in most patients with Cushing's disease. The patient in whom Cushing's disease cannot be differentiated from ectopic ACTH (e.g., particularly that caused by indolent carcinoid tumors) may need catheterization of the inferior petrosal sinuses (venous drainage of the anterior pituitary) and corticotropin-releasing hormone infusion to measure ACTH gradients in attempt to identify the pituitary as the source of ACTH (page 95). A chest CT or preferably magnetic resonance imaging searching for the small carcinoid tumor that may be producing ACTH and/or corticotropin-releasing hormone (mimicking Cushing's disease) should be considered.

Treatment

The treatment of Cushing's disease has already been discussed (page 96). The treatment of adrenal adenoma or carcinoma is by surgical adrenalectomy and even nephrectomy for the large and invasive adrenal carcinoma. Because removal of the tumor causing ectopic ACTH syndrome is rarely possible, treatment of the hypercortisolism with inhibitors of cortisol biosynthesis helps alleviate the weakness and hypokalemia. Three adrenal enzyme inhibitors are available for blocking steroidogenesis: ketoconazole (200–400 mg bid), aminoglutethimide (250 mg qid), and metyrapone (250–500 mg qid). All decrease cortisol production and are often used in combination for optimal results. Mitotane (o,p'DDD) is used to treat adrenal carcinoma that cannot be totally removed and metastatic adrenal carcinoma. Metastatic adrenal carcinoma has a poor prognosis with <50% survival at 3 years despite mitotane therapy. Patients with adrenal nodular dysplasia (pigmented micronodular dysplasia and macronodular hyperplasia) need bilateral adrenalectomy.

ADRENOCORTICAL INSUFFICIENCY

Inadequate adrenal function results from destruction of the cortex (primary adrenal insufficiency or Addison's disease) or from adrenocortical atrophy caused by ACTH deficiency (secondary adrenal insufficiency). In this latter circumstance mineralocorticoid function is preserved because the predominant regulator of aldosterone synthesis is the renin-angiotensin system not ACTH. There must be >90% destruction of the adrenal gland before Addison's disease is clinically apparent.

Eighty percent of Addison's disease is caused by autoimmune destruction of the adrenal glands, which is sometimes associated with other forms of polyglandular failure. Other causes of adrenal failure include granulomatous diseases (tuberculosis, histoplasmosis, sarcoidosis) and rarely infiltrative diseases (amyloid, lymphoma, hemochromatosis, adrenal leukodystrophy, and metastatic disease). Adrenal insufficiency is also found in some patients with AIDS. Adrenal crisis may be precipitated by any stress situation including fever, infection, radiographic studies, surgery, and so forth. One cause of adrenal insufficiency to be considered whenever a patient is taking anticoagulant medication is bilateral adrenal hemorrhage. This usually occurs 7–10 days after therapy is started and is associated with back pain. Female infants born with ambiguous genitalia and infants that fail to thrive may be adrenal insufficient because enzymes necessary to complete cortisol synthesis are lacking (congenital adrenal hyperplasia). The latent form (adult onset) of congenital adrenal hyperplasia is discussed on page 126.

Secondary adrenal atrophy caused by hypopituitarism has already been discussed (page 97). Exogenous glucocorticoids cause adrenal atrophy via suppression of ACTH. The same mechanism produces contralateral adrenal atrophy in cases of adrenal tumor causing Cushing's syndrome.

Clinical Presentation

Clinical features of chronic adrenal insufficiency include weakness, fatigue, and anorexia, which are invariably present, and gastrointestinal complaints of nausea, vague abdominal pain, and vomiting, which are seen less frequently. Salt craving is present in 20% of patients. Physical findings of weight loss, hyperpigmentation, and hypotension are generally found. The increased pigmentation results from increased melanin stimulation associated with raised ACTH levels. The hyperpigmentation is generalized but is accentuated in sun-exposed areas, the scrotum and perineum, nipple areola, skin creases, and areas subject to repeated trauma such as elbows, knuckles, and knees. These skin changes are not present in secondary adrenal insufficiency.

Some addisonian patients have stone-hard pinna caused by calcification of the auricular cartilage.

Infants and young children with adrenal insufficiency may present with failure to thrive, dehydration and salt wasting, and ambiguous genitalia in the female with masculinization. Decreased activity of
one of several adrenal enzymes leads to impaired cortisol production.
As a result, ACTH secretion increases and the adrenal enlarges,
hence, the name congenital adrenal hyperplasia. Precursor steroids
are shunted along accessory metabolic pathways leading to excessive
androgen production (21-hydroxylase and 11-hydroxylase deficiency)
and mineralocorticoid production (11-hydroxylase deficiency).

Laboratory

Low morning serum cortisol and elevated plasma ACTH character-
ize the laboratory findings of Addison's disease. Plasma cortisol fails to
rise after cosyntropin administration (page 11). Mineralocorticoid deficiency manifests as hyponatremia and hyperkalemia. An elevated
blood urea nitrogen reflects the prerenal azotemia of salt wasting and
volume contraction. Hypercalcemia is present in 6% of Addison's disease cases and remits with therapy. Fasting hypoglycemia may occur,
especially during crisis situations because of lack of glucocorticoid effect. A normochromic and normocytic anemia associated with an
eosinophilia is commonly present. If a macrocytic anemia is present,
one should suspect concomitant pernicious anemia.

Workup

Once the diagnosis of hypoadrenalism is considered, it is not difficult
to exclude or confirm. Any patient with unexplained weight loss
should be suspect for Addison's disease (other endocrine diseases to be
considered are thyrotoxicosis and diabetes mellitus). Are there symptoms compatible with hypoadrenalism (weakness, nausea, anorexia,
etc.)? Has the patient suddenly stopped taking glucocorticoids? Is
there a precipitating cause that has unmasked insufficient adrenal reserve (e.g., rifampim increases hepatic degradation of cortisol)? Is
there hyperpigmentation? Not all patients with chronic adrenal insufficiency are hyperpigmented. Because about 8% of addisonian patients do not have classical hyperpigmentation, one must rely on a
high index of suspicion to make the diagnosis (weakness and weight
loss are nearly always present). Often the addisonian patient presents
in adrenal crisis with hypotension, hypovolemia, abdominal pain that
may mimic an acute abdomen, and possibly fever. A tip-off to adrenal

insufficiency may come from the determination of serum cortisol during stress. Any subject with normal adrenal glands should have serum cortisol levels above 18 μg/dL during severe stress. Finding <u>hyponatremia</u>, <u>hyperkalemia</u>, and <u>azotemia</u> should suggest the possibility of hypoadrenalism. If the diagnosis of hypoadrenalism is suspected during a stress situation, one should obtain blood for cortisol and ACTH determinations and immediately begin intravenous Solu-Cortef along with normal saline as discussed on page 32. If the diagnosis is suspected in a nonacute situation or seems less likely, then provocative testing with a short course of ACTH is indicated (page 11).

Treatment

The treatment for adrenal crisis is discussed on page 32. The management during stress such as preparation for and during surgery is described on page 102. In the nonstressed situation, the euadrenal state is maintained with hydrocortisone (cortisol) 20–30 mg/day usually given bid, 10–20 mg at 7–8 AM, and 10 mg at 4–6 PM. An occasional patient may need 10 mg tid. Hydrocortisone is rapidly absorbed from the gut, and serum levels of cortisol peak after about 1 hour. Cortisone acetate may also be used for replacement. The dose is 25–37.5 mg/day given as 12.5–25 mg every morning and 12.5 mg every afternoon, a schedule identical to that for hydrocortisone. Cortisone acetate is absorbed just slightly slower than hydrocortisone and is converted to cortisol by numerous tissues. Cortisone acetate ($30–40/100 25-mg tablets) costs more than hydrocortisone ($12–15/100 20-mg tablets). Because the half-life of cortisol is 60–90 minutes, the serum cortisol falls to <3 μg/dL in the addisonian patient 6–7 hours after ingesting replacement doses. To evaluate whether replacement dosage is adequate, the clinician must assess the patient for signs and symptoms of inadequate or excessive steroid replacement. For the patient who is clinically under- or over-replaced with hydrocortisone or cortisone acetate, measurement of urine cortisol in patients on replacement is helpful to assure proper doses of glucocorticoids. Patients with hypopituitary hypoadrenalism need only glucocorticoid replacement since the renin-angiotensin system, which is the predominant regulator of mineralocorticoid metabolism, remains intact. Conversely, most patients with primary adrenal insufficiency need mineralocorticoid supplementation, although some patients do well on glucocorticoid therapy alone with liberal salt intake. <u>Fludrocortisone</u> (Florinef) is the mineralocorticoid preparation of choice because it is potent, has prolonged activity, and is less expensive than aldosterone or deoxycorticosterone. The dose of Florinef is 0.05–0.1 mg given as a single dose once a day or every other day as needed.

HYPERALDOSTERONISM

Excessive aldosterone production by autonomous functioning adrenal tissue (either an <u>adenoma</u> or <u>hypertrophied zona glomerulosa</u>) stimulates renal wasting of potassium and reabsorption of sodium. The clinical features of hyperaldosteronism reflect <u>volume expansion that leads to hypertension and hypokalemia</u>. Hyperaldosteronism (Conn's syndrome) is a rare cause of hypertension (much less than 1%). The key to the diagnosis is a suspicion of its possibility in any <u>hypokalemic hypertensive patient who is not taking diuretics</u>. The hypertension can be cured by surgery if an aldosterone-secreting adrenal adenoma is present. Aldosteronoma is more common in females (70% of the cases), whereas bilateral adrenal hypertrophy is seen with equal frequency in both sexes. Unfortunately hypertension caused by bilateral adrenal hypertrophy does not respond to adrenalectomy.

  <u>Most hyperaldosteronism is secondary</u>, i.e., reflecting a normal adrenal response to increased stimulation by the renin-angiotensin system. A decrease in effective blood volume (e.g., diuretic therapy, hepatic insufficiency, congestive heart failure, or nephrotic syndrome) or a decrease in renal perfusion (e.g., malignant hypertension or renal artery stenosis) stimulates renin production and angiotensin generation, leading to secondary hyperaldosteronism.

Workup

Any patient with hypertension and hypokalemia who is not taking diuretics must be evaluated for hyperaldosteronism. The symptoms are nonspecific and are related to hypokalemia: weakness, fatigue, and malaise. A history of medication use is important. Excessive ingestion of licorice (glycyrrhizinic acid found in licorice has mineralocorticoid activity) mimics hyperaldosteronism. Patients who chew tobacco that is heavily flavored with licorice may present with hypertension and hypokalemia. Plasma renin activity and urine aldosterone are low in these patients. Edema is absent in primary aldosteronism but is often present in secondary aldosteronism. Patients with hyperaldosteronism may not have hypokalemia, but I am not convinced that every hypertensive patient needs provocative testing such as captopril loading to identify these patients. Certainly, hypokalemia should be the "red flag" to think about hyperaldosteronism.

One should suspect hyperaldosteronism (primary or secondary) when there is hypokalemia and urinary potassium wasting (>30 mEq/24 hours). Almost all patients with primary aldosteronism have serum potassium levels below 4 mEq/L. With sodium intake restriction, hypokalemia and urine potassium wasting may not be present. The diagnosis of primary aldosteronism is made by demonstrating that the <u>renin-angiotensin system is suppressed and urine aldosterone is elevated</u> in the face of adequate sodium repletion. A normal or elevated plasma renin activity excludes primary hyperaldosteronism. A low plasma renin does not in itself make the diagnosis because 15–20% of the hypertensive population have suppressed renin activity. Thus, hypokalemia and low renin activity require that a 24-hour urine for aldosterone be collected. If the urine aldosterone is elevated, then one must determine whether the cause of the hyperaldosteronism is an adrenal adenoma or bilateral adrenal hyperplasia. <u>Localization with a high resolution CT scan is extremely helpful.</u> If the CT is positive for an adrenal mass, then surgery to remove the adenoma is required. If the CT scan is not diagnostic as it often is (these adenomas can be small), then studies measuring plasma aldosterone response to posture are indicated (page 22). Since patients with bilateral hyperplasia retain some responsiveness of the renin-angiotensin system, these patients raise their plasma aldosterone in response to erect posture after overnight recumbency; patients with adenoma have no such response and often have a paradoxical response with lowering of aldosterone levels to upright posture. Plasma aldosterone is measured while recumbent at 8 AM and at 12 noon after spending the morning walking about. If the plasma aldosterone does not rise (value after 4 hours of upright posture is identical to 8 AM recumbent value) and the CT scan is negative, then venous catheterization of the adrenals may demonstrate gradients of plasma aldosterone that localize the adenoma. These patients are given intravenous drip of ACTH (cosyntropin 0.25 mg in 250 mL normal saline) during the procedure so that plasma aldosterone-to-plasma cortisol ratios can be calculated and to ensure one is in the adrenal vein. Unfortunately the right adrenal vein often cannot be catheterized for technical and anatomical reasons.

Figure 14.2 diagrams an approach to evaluate the patient with hypertension and hypokalemia. An example of low renin and low aldosterone hypertension is Liddle's syndrome, a rare autosomal domi-

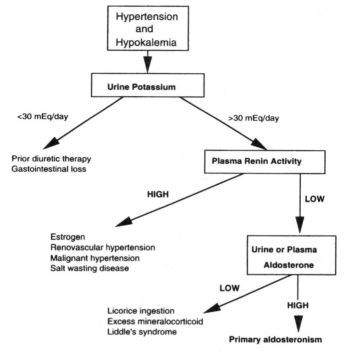

Figure 14.2.   Flow diagram to evaluate hypertension and hypokalemia.

nant disorder in which the renal tubule sodium channel is "locked in the open position," leading to excessive reabsorption of sodium and volume expansion and thus causing "pseudohyperaldosteronism."

Treatment

Treatment of aldosteronoma is by surgical removal of the adenoma. If the hyperaldosteronism is due to bilateral hyperplasia, spironolactone (100–400 mg/day) is prescribed since the hypertension responds poorly to surgery and since adrenalectomy leaves these patients dependent on exogenous steroids for the remainder of their lives. Spironolactone blocks the renal tubular effect of aldosterone and weakly inhibits aldosterone synthesis. Side effects of spironolactone at >100 mg/day are common and include gastrointestinal irritation, decreased libido, impotence, menstrual disturbances, and gynecomastia.

HYPOALDOSTERONISM

Hypoaldosteronism associated with hypocortisolism and salt wasting (Addison's disease) is discussed above. Because the primary regulator of aldosterone secretion is angiotensin II, any deficiency in the renin-angiotensin system may lead to hypoaldosteronism. Hyporeninemic hypoaldosteronism is caused by absent renin production by the kidney and is invariably seen in patients with renal insufficiency. Hyperkalemia and hyperchloremic acidosis along with azotemia are the biochemical findings. More than half the patients have diabetes mellitus, although many patients with AIDS have been found to have this syndrome of hyporeninemic hypoaldosteronism. The treatment is with fludrocortisone at higher doses (0.2 mg/day) than are normally required for Addison's disease. Better control of the blood sugar may ameliorate hyperkalemia in the diabetic patient.

PHEOCHROMOCYTOMA

Excessive production of catecholamines by tumors of chromaffin tissue of either the adrenal medulla or extra-adrenal sites leads to hypertension. The hypertension is sometimes episodic and severe, but sustained hypertension is present in most patients. Clinical features depend on the predominant catecholamine secreted. Norepinephrine-producing tumors are the most common and have hypertension as the primary manifestation. If these tumors also secrete significant amounts of epinephrine, then sweating, nervousness, and palpitations are present. A pure epinephrine-secreting tumor is rare and is marked by tachycardia, hypertension, and postural hypotension caused by epinephrine's effect on the β-adrenergic receptor causing vasodilation. Headache, excessive perspiration, and palpitations are frequent symptoms of pheochromocytoma. If a patient has none of the symptoms of this triad, there is a >99% probability that this patient does *not* have a pheochromocytoma. Paroxysmal attacks or spells may be provoked by exercise, postural change, abdominal palpation, urination (chromaffin tissue in the bladder wall is a rare site for tumor), or ingestion of some foods while being treated with monoamine oxidase inhibitors (certain cheeses and wines contain tyramine, which increases the release of catecholamines).

Workup

A family history of pheochromocytoma should be sought. Approximately 10% of the cases of pheochromocytoma are familial and occur as simple familial pheochromocytoma or as part of the multiple endocrine neoplasia syndrome (Type IIa or IIb). These patients are younger than the sporadic cases and often have bilateral adrenal and extra-adrenal sites of disease. Another autosomal dominant disorder associated with pheochromocytoma is von Hippel-Lindau disease (angioma of the retina, renal-cell carcinoma, pancreatic cysts, and epididymal cystadenoma). Neurofibromatosis and cafe-au-lait spots are associated with pheochromocytomas and should be sought by physical examination.

Pheochromocytoma cannot be diagnosed on clinical grounds alone. The suspicion of a catecholamine-producing tumor is raised in a hypertensive patient who has "spells" of sweating, headache, and palpitations. In fact, any patient with episodes of recurrent sweating, headache, or palpitations is a candidate for pheochromocytoma. The diagnosis requires biochemical evidence of increased catecholamine production. A 24-hour urine for catecholamines, metanephrines, or vanillylmandelic acid (a catechol breakdown product) should be ordered in such patients (page 23). Often two of these tests are ordered if the index of suspicion is very high to avoid missing the occasional patient who may not have an elevated value on one of these studies. Provocative testing with agents such as tyramine, histamine, or glucagon is not advised because the results are unreliable and the hazards related to the testing are substantial. Some endocrinologists use plasma catecholamine levels combined with clonidine suppression (normal and nonpheochromocytoma hypertensive patients decrease their plasma catecholamines in response to oral clonidine; pheo patients do not). There is considerable overlap between normal patients and those with pheochromocytoma, probably because the baseline plasma catecholamine levels vary so much. Urine studies, although not perfect (see "When, How, and What They Mean," Chapter 1), are more sensitive and specific than plasma catecholamine determinations. Localization of pheochromocytoma is facilitated by use of the CT scan. Metaiodobenzylguanidine (MIBG) is trapped by neural crest tissue. Scintiscan using radiolabeled 131-iodine MIBG helps localize disease in patients who have multiple pheochromocytomas or who have recurrent disease after surgery. The MIBG scan is positive in 80–90% of patients with a pheochromocytoma. In sporadic cases of pheochromocytoma the adrenal tumor is usually unilateral, but in familial disease these tumors are bilateral and often extra-adrenal. A chest X-ray should be performed before abdominal surgery to search for thoracic tumors. All patients with pheochromocytoma should have plasma calcitonin measured to identify those with multiple endocrine neoplasia type II. If medullary thyroid carcinoma is found, manage the pheochromocytoma first and later treat the thyroid malignancy.

Treatment

The treatment of pheochromocytoma is surgical removal of the cate-cholamine-producing tissue. Preoperative management requires α-adrenergic receptor blockade using phenoxybenzamine (Dibenzyline) in an initial dose of 10 mg tid. The dose is increased over several days (up to 40 mg tid) until the blood pressure stabilizes, symptoms abate, and hypovolemia remits. Urine determinations for vanillylmandelic acid and metanephrines are not affected by this medication. Propranolol is rarely used and then only after α-blockade is assured. Intravenous phentolamine (10–20 mg in 250 mL given as a microdrip and titrated to avoid irreversible shock) is used to treat acute hypertension episodes, although nitroprusside is an acceptable alternative. Intraoperative management requires expert anesthesia care. Propranolol and/or lidocaine is used to treat cardiac arrhythmias. The entire abdomen is explored, searching for multiple tumors along the aortic chain. Fortunately, <5% of pheochromocytomas are malignant. Patients with metastatic tumor can have their adrenergic symptoms controlled with phenoxybenzamine, but there is no effective chemotherapy for malignant pheochromocytoma. Large doses of 131-iodine MIBG can be used to treat metastatic pheochromocytoma.

INCIDENTAL ADRENAL MASS

With the advent of CT, many adrenal masses are serendipitously found. These incidental tumors are usually unilateral masses within the adrenal. They may be functioning or nonfunctioning tumors that histologically are benign or malignant. Nonfunctioning adrenal tumors are common. Clinically silent tumors occur in 1.4–8.7% of autopsied patients. Such tumors include benign cortical adenomas, cysts, myelolipomas, ganglioneuromas, hemorrhages, and granulomas. Malignant nonfunctioning masses include metastatic tumors and adrenal adenocarcinomas that are often bulky tumors (>6 cm). Functioning tumors include cortical adenomas that secrete cortisol (Cushing's syndrome), androgens (virilizing syndromes), aldosterone (Conn's syndrome), and medullary adenomas that secrete catecholamines (pheochromocytoma). Histologically, these tumors are generally benign.

Workup

The first question to address is whether the adrenal mass is metastatic disease. If the patient has known malignancy (e.g., breast or lung) and if the presence of adrenal metastases affects therapy, then CT guided biopsy is indicated. If the adrenal mass is truly incidental, the next question is whether the adrenal mass is a functioning or a nonfunctioning tumor. If it is a functioning endocrine tumor, surgical removal is necessary. The most common functioning tumor that is incidentally found is a pheochromocytoma. So all patients with an incidental adrenal mass need 24-hour urine collection for catecholamines, metanephrines, or vanillylmandelic acid. If the patient is hypertensive, then a serum potassium is obtained. If the potassium is <3.5 mEq/L, then get plasma renin level. If low, then perform urine aldosterone studies. If the patient clinically has any stigmata of Cushing's syndrome, then a 24-hour urine is obtained for free cortisol/17-hydroxycorticosteroid determinations. Use the data on Table 14.1 to exclude a functioning tumor.

If the tumor is nonfunctioning, use the following CT criteria to help determine whether the mass is benign or malignant. Three criteria are important: <u>size</u>, <u>contrast enhancement</u>, and <u>consistency</u>. Malignant adenocarcinomas are large (in six series, 105 out of 114 adenocarcinomas were ≥6 cm). Benign adenomas rarely get this size (three of 12,000 autopsies). <u>So any mass larger than 6 cm ought to be removed.</u> For most adrenal masses (i.e., nonfunctioning masses smaller than 6 cm), contrast enhancement and consistency help determine the probability of malignancy. Contrast enhancement is more often seen in malignant lesions. Benign adrenal lesions generally have a regular consistency (homogeneous appearance on CT), whereas malignant lesions show irregular consistency (hypodense and soft tissue mixed haphazardly). The CT is quite good in identifying benign cysts and myelolipomas, but the magnetic resonance imaging is more helpful in general. For example, metastatic disease and pheochromocytomas show greater T2 intensity compared with liver.

Table 14.1
Studies to Exclude Functioning Adrenal Incidentaloma

Possibility	Studies to Order
Pheochromocytoma	24-Hour urine for vanillylmandelic acid or metanephrine or catecholamines (get two different studies if patient hypertensive)
Cushing's syndrome	24-Hour urine for 17-OHCS/urine cortisol (dexamethasone study if urine abnormal or if Cushing's syndrome suspected clinically)
Hyperaldosteronism	Serum potassium on high sodium diet (≥200 mEq); if <3.5 or if patient is hypertensive, measure 24-hour urine aldosterone
Virilizing syndrome	24-Hour urine for 17-ketosteroids, 17-OHCS (serum testosterone, serum 17-OHCS if hirsute female; serum estrogen for feminized male or child)

OHCS, hydroxcorticosteroids.

Treatment

Small nonfunctioning benign-appearing lesions (e.g., 2.5 cm) should be followed with CT in 6–12 months to see if there is enlargement. Any increase in size dictates surgical removal. If the adrenal mass is unchanged in size over 1 year, it is unlikely to be a malignant lesion.

Suggested Readings

Aron DC, Tyrell JB, Fitzgerald PA, Findling JW, Forsham PH: Cushing's syndrome: problems in diagnosis. *Medicine* 60:24, 1981.

Baxter JD, Tyrell JB: The adrenal cortex. In Felig P, Baxter JD, Broadus AE, Frohman LA (eds): *Endocrinology and Metabolism*, ed 2. New York, McGraw-Hill, 1986, pp 511–650.

Burch WM: Urine-free cortisol determination: a useful tool in the management of chronic hypoadrenal states. *JAMA* 247:2002, 1982.

Copeland PM: The incidentally discovered adrenal mass. *Ann Intern Med* 98:940, 1983.

Cryer PE: Diseases of the sympathochromaffin system. In Felig P, Baxter JD, Broadus AE, Frohman LA (eds): *Endocrinology and Metabolism*, ed 2. New York, McGraw-Hill, 1986, pp 651–692.

Gill JR: Primary hyperaldosteronism: strategies for diagnosis and treatment. *Endocrinologist* 1:365, 1991.

Guerrero LA: Diagnostic and therapeutic approach to incidental adrenal mass. *Urology* 26:435, 1985.

Kaplan NM: Endocrine hypertension. In Wilson JD, Foster DW (eds): *Textbook of Endocrinology*, ed 7. Philadelphia, Saunders, 1985, pp 966–988.

Lacroix A, Bolte E, Tremblay J, et al: Gastric inhibitory polypeptide-dependent cortisol hypersecretion—a new cause of Cushing's syndrome. *N Engl J Med* 327:974, 1992.

Melby JC: Primary aldosteronism. *Kidney Int* 26:769, 1984.

Neumann HPH, Berger DP, Sigmund G, et al: Pheochromocytomas, multiple endocrine neoplasia type 2, and von Hippel-Landau disease. *N Engl J Med* 329:1531, 1993.

Orth DN: Differential diagnosis of Cushing's syndrome. *N Engl J Med* 325:957, 1991.

Ross NS, Aron DC: Hormonal evaluation of the patient with an incidentally discovered adrenal mass. *N Engl J Med* 323:1401, 1990.

Stein PP, Black HR: A simplified diagnostic approach to pheochromocytoma. *Medicine* 70:46, 1990.

Weinberger MH: Primary aldosteronism: diagnosis and differentiation of types. *Ann Intern Med* 100:300, 1984.

Chapter 15

The Weak and Tired Patient

Weakness, tiredness, fatigue, and lack of "energy" are frequent complaints voiced in the clinic or office of any physician. The nonspecificity of such complaints opens a Pandora's box of possible diagnoses. To make any sense of these symptoms, they must be integrated with other symptoms and physical signs. Onset and duration of symptoms, associated pain, weight change, fever, and medications are points that must be known. Important differential diagnoses that should be part of the thought process during the interview include anemia, cancer, renal or hepatic insufficiency, systemic infection, pulmonary disease, congestive heart failure, arthritides, diabetes mellitus, thyroid disease, and drugs (including alcohol).

Often the clinician must assess whether the tired and weak patient has a "metabolic" problem. This patient may have seen several other physicians seeking help for the fatigue and weakness. Although in most cases the asthenia cannot be attributed to a specific endocrine abnormality, these patients deserve the benefit of an honest attempt to address their problem. It is all too easy to make a premature diagnosis before actually hearing the patient out when she or he presents self-referred for "hypoglycemia" or with "maladie du petit papier." A thorough, unhurried interview by a sympathetic clinician may find a problem missed by others. The importance of an open mind, good history taking, and complete physical examination cannot be overemphasized in dealing with the weak and tired patient.

A logical approach to the weak, tired, dizzy, and gassy patient from the endocrine viewpoint is to ask specific questions that relate to possible hormone causes. Representative questions for several hormones and hormone-secreting organs follow.

PITUITARY HORMONE

Are menses regular? Regular intervals of menstruation make hypopituitarism unlikely. Is there galactorrhea that may be related to a prolactinoma? Has there been acral growth? Has there been a change in visual acuity? Loss of vision is relatively common with large pituitary tumors.

ADRENAL HORMONE

Is there hyperpigmentation? Chronic primary adrenal insufficiency leads to darkening of skin, particularly in areas of repeated pressure. Is there any weight loss, nausea, vomiting, or syncope? Is there evidence of hypercortisolism? Episodes of tachycardia, headaches, and sweating are suggestive of pheochromocytoma.

THYROID HORMONE

Is there a change in neck size or shape to suggest a goiter? What is the patient's room temperature preference; 60, 70, or 80°F? Preferring 60° suggests hyperthyroidism; preferring 80° suggests possible hypothyroidism. Are there other symptoms and signs of hypothyroidism (e.g., hoarseness, muscle cramps, sleepiness, dry skin, puffy facies, delayed relaxation time of deep tendon reflexes) or hyperthyroidism (e.g., nervousness, anxiety, weight loss despite good appetite, increased sweating, smooth skin, tremor, proptosis, tachycardia)? Is there neck pain?

PARATHYROID HORMONE

Has there ever been thyroid or neck surgery? Surgical hypoparathyroidism is the most common cause of hypocalcemia. Kidney stones, polyuria, and constipation indicate hypercalcemia.

PANCREAS

Is there nocturia? Is there noctidipsia? Diabetes mellitus with glycosuria with osmotic diuresis should considered. Has weight changed? Weight loss despite increased appetite also suggests diabetes mellitus. Are there symptoms compatible with fasting hypoglycemia (e.g., mental confusion, "glassy" eyes, and sweating that are relieved by food)?

TESTES

Is there impotence? Impotence caused by primary hypogonadism responds to androgen replacement.

OVARIES

Is there premature menopause? Is there amenorrhea or galactorrhea compatible with a prolactinoma?

DISCUSSION

More often than not, the patient who presents with weakness has chronic fatigue, is a female between 20 and 50 years old, and frequently has the idea that something like hypoglycemia "must" be the cause of the weakness and lack of energy. The history may be reiterated from a sheet of paper "so I won't forget anything." Social and interpersonal relationships are often a source of unadmitted conflict. Anxiety and/or stress is the most common diagnosis, yet this should be a diagnosis of exclusion made after a careful review of the history, physical examination, and laboratory studies. Specific laboratory studies are warranted as deemed necessary by the history and physical examination and may be needed to assure the patient that nothing has been overlooked.

LABORATORY STUDIES

Screening laboratory studies using automated techniques are useful. These include complete blood count; urine analysis; serum sodium, potassium, bicarbonate, chlorine, blood urea nitrogen; plasma glucose; serum calcium; serum glutamic-oxaloacetic transaminase, serum glutamic-pyruvic transaminase, bilirubin, and alkaline phosphatase activity.

Thyroid (pages 3–5) and adrenal (page 11) functions can be assessed if necessary.

Although postprandial reactive hypoglycemia exists, it is very difficult to separate this condition from pseudohypoglycemia or nonhypoglycemia, as discussed in Chapter 4. There is no good test to confirm this "entity." If one orders a oral glucose tolerance test, then be prepared to defend the results (either negative or positive) to the patient.

Absent menses in a women of childbearing years can be due to pregnancy, which must be excluded. Serum prolactin is obtained when there is a history of amenorrhea or oligomenorrhea and/or galactorrhea.

Serum testosterone and gonadotropins (follicle-stimulating hormone and luteinizing hormone) are indicated if hypogonadism is a possibility.

If the clinical index for suspicion of any endocrine diagnosis is low and laboratory results do not indicate a specific problem, then be honest with the patient. Give your opinion, but remember the 15th century proverb that summarizes the purpose of medicine: **"To cure sometimes, to relieve often, to comfort always."**

Index

Page numbers in *italics* denote figures; those followed by "t" denote tables.